The Coalbrookdale

The Coalbrookdale Doctors

A Family Practice in Shropshire, 1770-1870

Richard Moore

YOUCAXTON PUBLICATIONS

OXFORD & SHREWSBURY

Copyright © Richard Moore 2014

The Author asserts the moral right to
be identified as the author of this work.

ISBN 978-1-909644-30-4
Printed and bound in Great Britain.
Published by Richard Moore 2014

All rights reserved. No part of this publication may be reproduced,
stored in a retrieval system, or transmitted in any form or by
any means, electronic, mechanical, photocopying, recording or
otherwise, without the prior permission of the publisher.

This book is sold subject to the condition that it shall not, by way of
trade or otherwise, be lent, resold, hired out or otherwise circulated
without the publisher's prior consent in any form of binding or cover
other than that in which it is published and without a similar condition
including this condition being imposed on the subsequent purchaser.

Contents

Preface	viii
Acknowledgements	xi
The Coalbrookdale Doctors: the Historical Context	1
Benjamin in Coalbrookdale: Surgeon-Apothecary	14
William	31
Edward	50
William and Edward	70
Plates	89
Edward in London	98
Edward in the Practice	116
Benjamin in London	134
Reform and Partnership	154
Finale	172
Bibliography	183
Chronology	187
Index	193

Plates

1. *Map of Coalbrookdale, from The Tithe Map 1849*, Shropshire Archives, page 90.

2. *Coalbrookdale at Night*, by Philip James de Loutherburg, 1801, Science Museum, London page 91.

3. *Coalbrookdale Works, Fire Engine and Mill-pond, by R. R. Angerstein, 1755,* Ironbridge Gorge Museum Trust Collection, page 92.

4. *The Iron Bridge*, by William Williams, 1779, Ironbridge Gorge Museum Trust Collection, page 92.

5. *A View of the Upper Works at Coalbrookdale*, by François Vivares, 1758, Ironbridge Gorge Museum Trust Collection, page 93.

6. *An afternoon view of Coalbrookdale*, by William Williams, 1771, Shropshire Council, Shropshire Museum, page 93.

7. *The Dance of Death: the Apothecary*, by T. Rowlandson, 1816, Wellcome Library, London, page 94.

8. *A surgeon bleeding the arm of a young woman,* by T. Rowlandson, 1784, Wellcome Library, London, page 94.

9. *A Man-Mid-Wife, a newly discovered animal not known before*, by Isaac Cruikshank, 1793, Wellcome Library, London, page 95.

10. *A collection of Laennec's stethoscopes, early 19th Century*, Wellcome Library, London, page 96.

11. *Reconstruction of Trevithick's steam locomotive, built in 1803,* Ironbridge Gorge Museum Trust Collection, page 96.

12. *Rose Hill in 2014*, author's photograph, page 97.

Preface

Every reader of *The Coalbrookdale Doctors* may be forgiven for being alarmed at some of the treatments that were once commonly practised by medical men. My forebear, Ann Sorton, was bled twice, alas, to no avail. The reader must be careful not to condemn those of the Eighteenth Century with the accumulated knowledge of the Twenty-First Century. One may observe and then give heartfelt thanks for the wonders of modern medicine.

Dr. Richard Moore is well aware of this dichotomy and has skilfully placed the lives and work of the Coalbrookdale doctors in the context in which each one lived, covering both social and medical aspects. There are fascinating details about their patients and the prevailing poverty when trade was bad, causing difficulties in paying for medical treatment. Interestingly, Benjamin Wright also helped finance life in the Dale by putting his name to Bills of Exchange, an unusual activity for a doctor.

There were few effective medicines when Benjamin Wright arrived in Coalbrookdale in 1775 as apothecary-surgeon and, when ill, many people used herbal concoctions that were unlikely to benefit them. Roads were bad and the doctors went on horseback to visit many of their patients. Their horses were not fast ones and journeys were sometimes as much as ten miles or more. Times were hard.

We must remember that, in the Eighteenth Century, there was an enormous increase in the use of coal by the various industries throughout the whole district. The silica in coal dust made coal more dangerous to both workers and those who lived nearby than did the use of charcoal.

In Coalbrookdale alone there were two blast-furnaces using coke as fuel and each of these furnaces needed twice as much fuel as

PREFACE

a charcoal-smelting furnace. From 1742 there was a Newcomen steam-engine to pump the water back to the furnace pool. These operations were continuous.

In the late 1770s Charles Hornblower of the Coalbrookdale Company listed the operations required for the charging of a furnace. These include:

> The ore is calcined (or roasted) in heaps of 1000 tons. 200 tons of coal or less wd *(sic)* burn 1000 tons of Iron Stone, which is done by laying the Coal about 13 inches thick on the ground and covering it with Iron Stone. If the heap is made thicker it is useful to throw a little slack or small coal into the Heap of Stone. This quantity will require 3 Weeks to calcine a whole heap... The Coal is burned into Coak *(sic)* in heaps of about 9 or 10 Tons which is done in 36 hours...

There were important advances in medicine in the century covered by the doctors in Coalbrookdale such as the discovery by Jenner in 1796 of vaccination to prevent smallpox, the invention of the stethoscope in 1816 (published 1819) and the discovery of anaesthetics in the 1840s. These laid the foundation of modern diagnostic medicine and surgery and equally as important was the progress being made in training doctors. Benjamin Wright's training had been sketchy in comparison with that of his grandson Benjamin who started his studies in 1835 and spent some time at the newly-founded King's College, London. Also during this period, *The Lancet* and the forerunner of *The British Medical Journal* were established and professional regional gatherings were organised. That in Shrewsbury was started in 1838.

The grandsons of Benjamin Wright, Edward and Benjamin Edwards, were qualified by public and increasingly rigorous examinations. The old system of apothecary-surgeon had ended with the deaths of their father and grandfather. Dr. Richard Moore declares clearly and confidently that there was now a new medical profession, that ... 'this was the dawn of the medical profession that we have today ... the future of the profession was bright'.

It gives me much pleasure to commend this book that describes so well the transition in Coalbrookdale from the work of apothecary-surgeons to doctors '... at the dawn of the modern medical profession'.

Michael Darby

Acknowledgements

The inspiration for this book is the correspondence between members of the Wright and Edwards family written when the youngest generation, Edward and Benjamin Edwards, were in London studying to be doctors. Additional research into the family and their environment in the industrial village of Coalbrookdale has been done. Edward and Benjamin wrote home about their own activities and public events in the capital, and various members of the family replied with news of family matters, their medical business and local affairs. The Wright and Edwards family were neighbours of the Darbys and friendly with them, which is why the letters found their way into the possession of Lady Rachel Labouchere, a descendant of Abraham Darby I (1678-1717), and thence into the Shropshire Archives. They have been used in other accounts of Coalbrookdale to illustrate occasional events, including V.A.C. Gatrell's learned discussion of the curious medico-legal case of Elizabeth Cureton, but this is the first use of these letters in the parallel contexts of the developing medical profession and the industrial, social and political changes of the eighteenth and nineteenth centuries.

This account of three generations of a family of doctors traces the development of general medical practice over one hundred years in the late Eighteenth to the mid-Nineteenth Centuries. It starts with an outline of an early form of general medical practitioner, the apothecary-surgeon, and progresses to illustrate the work of local doctors who laid the foundations of the general practice system we have today. Thus it offers an insight into a period of history in which various kinds of doctor began to establish themselves in a scientifically educated and legally regulated profession, and sought to exclude untrained — and therefore supposedly unsafe — competitors. The account is set in the context of the scientific and political developments of the period, which were of unprecedented extent and rapidity, and laid the foundations of the modern 'global village'.

I am much indebted to many people connected with the characters in the story. Three descendants of Benjamin Wright, the first Coalbrookdale doctor, have generously made available material from their own family history research; they are Sue Hemming, Pam Jones and Julie Wright. Their enthusiastic interest in the story of their forbear Benjamin Wright, and their many-times-removed cousins in the Edwards family has been a great help and inspiration to me. I am very grateful to Michael Darby, contemporary descendant of the Darby family, the well-known ironfounders featured in the story, who has given me invaluable advice about his forebears as well as technical information about the iron industry. He has also authorised payment of the fees for using the Ironbridge Gorge Museum's images from the Quaker Book Fund. I thank Mr and Mrs Coxson, present owners of the one-time home of the Edwards family, who kindly allowed me to visit their house and take photographs of it. I also thank Mrs Darlington, church warden of Coalbrookdale church, and Dr Andrew Pattison for helpful comments on an early draft.

I am much indebted to V.A.C. Gatrell for his account of the Cureton case in which Edward Edwards played a significant role. The help which I have received from Shropshire Archives, the Ironbridge Gorge Museum Trust Library, The Wellcome Institute and the many other sources listed in the Bibliography is very gratefully acknowledged. If any people or organisations who have been of assistance have been omitted the fault is mine alone.

Chapter 1
The Coalbrookdale Doctors: the Historical Context

Benjamin Wright was born in 1745 into a changing world. As he was growing up, old certainties were being challenged everywhere. At home, new ideas in agriculture, commerce and politics were changing social structures while, overseas, merchant adventurers were exploring the world. Radical thinkers were challenging the hegemony of monarchies and aristocracies and proclaiming the benefits of democracy. More belligerently, in America the British colonists were fighting their French and Spanish rivals before rebelling against their King

The principal characters in this book, Benjamin Wright, his son-in-law William Edwards and his grandsons Edward and Benjamin Edwards, were real people who experienced both the thrills and threats of those exciting times. They were doctors in the village of Coalbrookdale in Shropshire, which in 1837 was described as 'the most extraordinary district in the world'[1] because of the major advances in the manufacture and use of iron that were made there as the Industrial Revolution gathered pace. Benjamin Wright set up his business as surgeon-apothecary in 1770, treating the sick and injured, delivering babies and selling medicines, though in the usually vain hope that they would be effective. The business, later to be renamed 'the practice', was continued by his family for nearly a hundred years. At the same time, a new era of power, transport, travel, comfort, communication, speed and noise began to merge the self-contained and slowly-changing communities of the world into

---

1 Hulbert, Charles, *The History and Description of the County of Salop*, p. 348, Published by the author, 1837.

what now seems to be an ever-changing global village. Progress may appear faster today than ever before but the changes experienced by those who lived between 1750 and 1850 were arguably even more extreme. It was an exciting time to be alive.

Life in Britain was simple when Benjamin was born. Most people lived and died within a few miles of their childhood homes and, though some were rich from inheritance or became wealthy through trade and enterprise, standards of living for the majority were low and often bleak. Most houses could hardly keep out the winter cold and were dimly lit by feeble candles and their sanitary systems were malodorously foul. For many people, the diet was plain and meat was a rarity. Disease was common and lives were short, even for those who survived the perils of birth and infancy. The everyday things of Twenty-First Century life — warm homes, electric power, transport, travel and communication — were not even the stuff of dreams.

Benjamin did not stay where he was born, however, because, as the fourth of the seven sons and one daughter of Benjamin and Mary Wright, farmers of Tattenhall in Cheshire, he had to find his own living. He was apprenticed to a surgeon-apothecary in Broseley, Shropshire, to learn that trade, exchanging rural Cheshire for the clamorous world of industry and commerce. In Benjamin's youth there were no newspapers or broadcasts to tell him of the political upheavals and wars in which Britain, France and Spain engaged in a global struggle to defend their interests. In America the British colonists who sought religious and political freedom fought for their new homeland against their French and Spanish rivals, threw off the shackles of taxation without representation and declared themselves to be a new nation. Despite Britain losing the consequent War of Independence, the many successes of the Royal Navy ensured the security for Britain of the prosperous trade routes to the West Indies, Africa and India that made Britain the richest nation in the world. The fortunes of its citizens were soon to prosper as never before.

While all this was happening abroad, Benjamin Wright established himself as the surgeon-apothecary of Coalbrookdale. In 1766, at the age of twenty-one, having served his time as apprentice, he would have been free to work on his own account. His marriage in 1768 to Frances, daughter of the ironmaster, John Guest of Broseley, suggests that he was soon in a favourable position to start his own business. Broseley was thriving from the rapidly developing iron industry, and the ironmasters of the area would have known each other well. Many of the leaders of the new industrial and commercial enterprises were members of the Society of Friends, or Quakers, which was also well-supported in Cheshire and the north west of England where Benjamin was brought up. Through marriage into the Guest family he would have been introduced to the Darby family who were leading Quakers in Coalbrookdale on the other side of the River Severn and proprietors of the successful Coalbrookdale Company. He was probably encouraged or even supported by Darby to open a new business for the benefit of the increasing number of workers in Coalbrookdale. Benjamin's patronage by Abraham Darby seems all the more likely because in the early years of their marriage he and Frances lived in The Grange (later called Rosehill in what is now Darby Road) which had been acquired by Darby in 1760. He probably had his apothecary's shop in the house — it is certainly large enough.[2] It was here that Benjamin and Frances raised their family: Mary, the oldest, was born in 1770 and was followed in the next seventeen years by four more daughters and three sons.

The apothecary's trade was a very old one. It began as an offshoot of the grocery trade specialising in the sale of plant-based medicines along with perfumes, wigs and other personal items. It had a reputation for superstition and some practitioners may even have encouraged a sense of impenetrable mystery to offset the ineffectiveness of their remedies.

---

[2] Notes on Rosehill House and Benjamin Wright, Ironbridge Gorge Museum Trust. The house is now part of the museum and is open to the public.

As reason replaced superstition during the eighteenth century, this unfavourable attitude gradually changed to an expectation of benefit. Prints of apothecaries' shops emphasise the inscrutability of their craft: dried crocodile and lizard skins hang above benches laden with curious apparatus; customers wait to be served by the well-dressed proprietor; and in the background an overworked apprentice grinds the *materia medica* or distills the potions. At the time that Benjamin started his business, medical care was beginning to abandon mystery and superstition in favour of careful observation and scientific reason though the process was slow. There has always been a demand to cure disease, so with rising national prosperity and a more rational approach many apothecaries became so financially successful that in a society very conscious of class they were able to lift themselves out of trade and into the ranks of the minor gentry, or even higher.

In 1789, while Benjamin and Frances's children were still young, social and political forces in France exploded into bloody revolution and war. In Coalbrookdale, however, it was not war but the clamour and fire of industry which disturbed the peace, because there the industrial revolution was in full flow. Coalbrookdale's most famous achievement in Benjamin's time was the construction of the world's first cast iron bridge, built in the 1770s to enable heavy goods to cross the turbulent river Severn and also to demonstrate the strength of the Coalbrookdale Company's material, produced by a new and improved method. Another 'first' was John Wilkinson's iron boat, *The Trial*. Though sceptics said it 'would not swim', its launch was witnessed by a large crowd and saluted by firing a 32-pounder canon and, according to Wilkinson, it 'answered all his expectations ... and convinced 999 out of 1000 unbelievers'.[3] It was the first of millions of iron-hulled ships.

Such was the prosperity of the area, especially of the Coalbrookdale Company, that Benjamin prospered too and was able to buy his own

---

3 Randall, J., *History of Madeley including Ironbridge, Coalbrookdale and Coalport*, Wrekin Echo Office, Madeley, 1880, p. 108.

small estate in the Dale. By 1794, he and his family had moved into a newly-built house called Greenbank. The children were between seven and twenty years old, though one boy had died young. It should have been a joyful move but hard times were to come. The family had only just moved to their new home when Benjamin fell ill and, within a few months, was dead. The widowed Frances left Greenbank, which was let, and moved with the younger girls into a smaller house. The oldest daughter Mary married, and the two surviving boys, Peter at seventeen and Benjamin fifteen, were able to earn their livings in the Dale. Before long, the second daughter Elizabeth married William Edwards, apothecary, who took over the business. William and Elizabeth moved to a house confusingly called Rose Hill near to but not the same as the Rosehill where Benjamin and Frances had lived. The new Rose Hill became the Edwards family's home, and William opened a shop there from which to conduct his business.

But all was not well in the wider world. In the 1790s, France descended into revolutionary chaos and another twenty years of war began in Europe. The demands for freedom and equality in France had sympathetic supporters in England, such as the poet William Wordsworth — 'Bliss was it in that dawn to be alive' he wrote in his youthful enthusiasm.[4] In the face of long military campaigns abroad and the threat of invasion at home calls for reform were resisted until after 1815 when peace was secured, although the political uncertainty depressed manufacturing industries, particularly in Coalbrookdale. (In some places the iron industry was able to capitalise on the demand for armaments, but the Darbys, proprietors of the Coalbrookdale Company, were Quakers and therefore pacifists who would not participate in the manufacture of military materials.) In the post-war years there was a resurgence of social and industrial unrest as long-suppressed demands for reform were heard again. Life in the Dale was hard and, to add to the economic troubles, the summer crops failed

---

4 William Wordsworth, *The French Revolution, as it appeared to an Enthusiast.*

and the winters were severe, causing periods of famine amongst the poor. For them, and even the not-so-poor, the excitement of progress turned to the despair of depression.

Despite the economic depression, these were times of unprecedented progress: as peace continued, developments in science, trade, industry, travel and communication foreshadowed the world we know today and, in medicine, changing social attitudes and the gradual adoption of scientific methods began to shape the modern medical profession. This brought about the reform of medical education which changed from an uncoordinated system of apprenticeships to a science-based curriculum taught in formal medical schools. William's business survived the economic depression and, as soon as his oldest son, Edward, was fourteen he became William's apprentice. In Benjamin and William's time apprentices in the apothecary's trade studied botany, elementary chemistry, doggerel Latin and how to prepare medicines. They were commonly exploited as cheap labour, but there was little supervision and no test of competence at the end of training. By contrast, Edward and his contemporaries, though continuing with botany and *materia medica* also studied the newly-discovered elements in chemistry and, above all, human anatomy and pathology.

The end of the Eighteenth and early years of the Nineteenth Centuries, during which William and Edward were the Coalbrookdale doctors, was a fertile period of scientific discovery, typified by the work of three men who were giants of this age of discovery. Humphry Davy (1778-1829) received a rudimentary scientific education as apprentice to an apothecary-surgeon. Later he experimented with gases, including chlorine and nitrous oxide, the so-called 'laughing gas', and identified potassium, sodium and calcium. His distinguished career culminated in his election as President of the Royal Society and being created Baronet. Michael Faraday (1791-1867), the son of a blacksmith, also had an elementary education, was then apprenticed to a bookbinder and, like Davy, extended his learning whenever he could. He became the assistant to Davy at the Royal Institution and was later appointed Director of its laboratory. He is famous for his work in electromagnetism, especially the demonstration that an electric current passing through a magnetic field can generate motion — the original electric motor. The Scotsman James Watt (1736-1819) developed steam engines that were far more powerful than the earlier engines of Savery and Newcomen. It is noteworthy that these sons of artisans were resourceful men and did not have a privileged education. It was their genius, curiosity and determination that led them to experiment, learn and invent.

Advances in science inevitably affected the medical profession, which responded to the social and scientific changes around it. Doctors of all types who had adopted the new rational methods faced increasing competition from a host of untrained opportunists and quacks who flooded the market with remedies of their own invention. This seriously affected the financial security of those who had gone to the expense of acquiring proper training and experience. In an attempt to overcome this opposition the apothecary-surgeons demanded that parliament should protect them from unfair competition, which resulted in the Apothecaries Act of 1815. This Act instituted the first examination to demonstrate the competence of medical students at the end of their training. For the general public the Act identified for the first time a group of people who could claim to be properly qualified to practice medicine, but for individuals such as Edward it prolonged and increased the cost of their education. Even so, as soon as his father could afford it, Edward went to London to study and took the new examination. On his return to Coalbrookdale he worked with his father for fifteen years until 1827, when William died. This left Edward to run the practice on his own with the help of an assistant, and at times an apprentice also, until his younger brother Benjamin was old enough to join the business. As well as his own practical experience as an apprentice he had to study for the examination, which by now required spending two years or more in London. He went to London in 1837, returning during the vacations to work in the practice. He finally came back to Coalbrookdale in 1839 to join his brother in a partnership that lasted for thirty years until their retirement in the 1870s. During that time the re-organisation of the medical profession gathered pace, culminating, in 1858, in the Medical Act which set up the Medical Register of medical practitioners who had been appropriately trained. Medical practice by those who were ineligible to register was made illegal, a measure intended to prevent practice by quacks and charlatans which was not entirely successful.

This summary of the historical context would not be complete without a brief description of Coalbrookdale, because the production and manufacturing of iron was the basis of the doctors' livelihood and it did not always prosper. Although in its industrial heyday Coalbrookdale was described as 'the most extraordinary place in the world', at one time it had been one of the most tranquil. It is a valley some mile and a half long that cuts through a high plateau to join the larger gorge of the River Severn on its way to the sea. In medieval times it was steep-sided and well wooded with a small but constant stream running through it. But that was its undoing, because beneath the limestone surface lay deposits of coal and iron, and the stream was a source of power for exploiting these minerals. Since the Twelfth Century Coalbrookdale had belonged to St Milburga's Priory at Much Wenlock, a few miles away on the other side of the Severn. In 1332 one Walter de Cladbrook was granted permission to 'dig for coals at Brockholes', on the eastern side of the Dale.[5] It is tempting to think that the Dale is named after Cladbrook, or perhaps from coal, the 'black gold' that lies beneath its slopes. But as early as 1250 it was already known as 'Cold Brook Valley', and the word 'cold' has since become corrupted into 'coal'.[6]

---

5 Randall, J., *History of Madeley*, p 59.

6 *Concise Oxford Dictionary of Place-Names*, Oxford University Press, 1960, quoting Eyton, R.W., *Antiquities of Shropshire*, London, 1854-60.

Since the Iron Age more than 2,500 years ago, iron had been extracted from its ore by heating it in 'bloomeries', pits in the ground covered by a clay or stone chimney. The iron which separated out from the ore could be cast into shapes to form relatively small objects or 'forged' by being repeatedly hammered which made it strong enough for use as tools or swords. In Britain the industry flourished in many places, especially in Sussex where wood for making charcoal was abundant, but in Shropshire also. As demand grew the small and inefficient bloomeries were replaced by brick towers that could contain much more ore and in which the fuel burned at a greater heat because air was 'blasted' into it by water-powered bellows.[7]

Coalbrookdale was an ideal place for smelting iron because there were abundant supplies of iron ore, low-sulphur coal suitable for making coke and of limestone to use as flux in the furnaces. A blast furnace had been built in Coalbrookdale as early as 1658 and was operated successfully until 1704 when it was destroyed by an explosion. It lay derelict until 1709, when Abraham Darby repaired it and brought it into production again.[8] In the following decades successive generations of the Darby family and their business partners increasingly used coke for smelting, which, though made by partially burning coal, contains fewer impurities and thus produces a stronger and more versatile metal.

Coalbrookdale lies in the parish of Madeley, a medieval village that grew in size as workers came to work in the new industries. It is now part of Telford new town though the Dale itself has not been built over. In the mid-Eighteenth Century about four thousand people in some nine hundred families lived in Madeley. At the first census in 1801 the population had risen slightly to 4,750 and by 1871 had

---

[7] Watts, S., 'Shifnal Iron Accounts, 1583-90' in *Shropshire Historical Documents, a Miscellany*, Centre for Local History, University of Keele, 2000, pp12-3.

[8] Raistrick, A., *Dynasty of Iron Founders, the Darbys and Coalbrookdale*, Sessions Book Trust, in association with Ironbridge Gorge Museum Trust, 1989, pp 23, 30.

doubled to 9,500. Not all these people lived in Coalbrookdale itself, but these figures show the rapidity of industrial growth in this part of Shropshire.[9] Progress was bought at a price. The destruction of the natural beauty and ancient tranquillity of the Dale did not pass without notice. In her poem *Colebrook Dale,* the Romantic poet Anna Seward (1747-1809) commented on the desecration of this once beautiful place by fiery industry, bemoaning the violation of its peace: –

> Tribes fuliginous invade
> The soft, romantic, consecrated scenes;
> Haunt of the wood nymph, who with airy step,
> In times long vanished ranged through thy pathless groves.[10]

She speaks of countless fires with 'umber'd flames' and columns of 'thick sulphureous smoke' that rise like 'palls over the dead', polluting the air and staining the 'glassy water'. She prays that, in future, manufacturing cities elsewhere such as 'resounding' Birmingham and 'grim' Wolverhampton which were 'careless of art and knowledge', would get their all-polluting metal from some other source and let this lovely Dale recover its beauty. Though Seward's diatribe is overtly romantic, she was not alone in her comments. In his *Tours of England* of 1776, Arthur Young (1741-1820) regretted the loss of the Dale's sylvan charms but felt a mixture of wonder and horror in the scene he found.

> Coalbrookdale itself is a very romantic spot ... a winding glen between two hills ... all thickly covered with beautiful sheets of hanging woods ... too beautiful to be in unison with that variety of horrors art has spread

---

9   Randall, J., *History of Madeley,* p 166.

10 From *The Poetical Works of Anna Seward, Vol 2.* 'Fuliginous' = 'sooty', OED Online edition.

below. The noise of the forges, the flames bursting from the furnaces ... with the burning of the coal and the smoak *(sic)* of the lime kilns are altogether sublime[11].

It was the Age of the Sublime and the Picturesque, so artists came to paint these fiery scenes. William Williams's view from the top of the Dale, of 1771, shows a well-wooded valley, the outline of the ironmaster's houses and the River Severn in the distance. The only hint of industry is a column of smoke rising gently in the still air. The scene painted by George Robertson (1724-1788) is more 'fuliginous', to use Seward's word: smoke erupts from blazing furnaces while the Severn is crowded with barges and overshadowed by towering hills. By far the most dramatic is that of Philip de Loutherbourg (1740-1812). In his vivid 1801 painting of the Madeley Wood furnace, vast flames light the night sky, gauntly silhouetting the factory buildings. A team of horses struggles to pull a heavy load along an ill-made road between heaps of industrial detritus. To some it speaks of a new and mighty age, but to the people of that time it probably conjured an image of Hell. So much attention was drawn to the wonders of Coalbrookdale by poets and artists, whether by shock or sorrow, that tourists flocked to see it for themselves, with varying results. One contemporary but anonymous writer said that:

> Within 4 or 5 miles [of Coalbrookdale] there are upwards of thirty blast furnaces, making on average upward of fifty thousand tons of cast metal, the greater part of which is converted into wrought and malleable iron. The works of the vicinity are frequently visited by numbers of people of most ranks & stations in life, who seem much astonished by the extensiveness of the Manufactory and the regularity with which it is

---

11 Young, A., *Tours of England.*

conducted, oft expressing surprise that a situation so passing excellent should be fixed upon for the seat of so large a Manufactory.[12]

This writer said Coalbrookdale itself was a 'romantic spot' where among 'oak and birch woods ... the workmen's houses and gardens [provide] a pretty appearance', but also reported the less happy experience of a gentleman who sent his servant in advance. The man arrived at night without knowing what to expect and found the whole place 'a deluge of flames'. Terrified by what he saw, he returned to his master and reported that 'the whole valley was on fire, and begged him to proceed no further'.

The Industrial Revolution could not be halted by poets, artists or the fears of a horrified manservant. It changed the nation, indeed the whole world: people moved from country into the growing towns to find work; new wealth raised living standards and increased the demand for goods that in turn stimulated manufacture and employment. With faster travel, people and goods could reach more distant places and this began to unite the nation. The mail coach, railways and the penny post made long-distance communication feasible for all. In 1800 London was more than a day's journey from Shropshire by uncomfortable, sluggish horse-drawn coaches or carts over sometimes impassable roads, but by the 1850s it could be reached comfortably by train in four hours. Education became more widely available, literacy increased and science and literature flourished. In government, oligarchy gave way to democracy; in towns gas lamps lit the streets at night. But not all change was good or worthy. Poverty and misery were widespread and housing, though grand for some, was miserable for others; fatal epidemics were frequent; it was a man's world in which women generally took second place. For shame, the drive for profit exploited

---

12 SA 1987/64/6, *A Sketch of Coalbrookdale*, manuscript, unsigned and undated.

men, women and even children in injurious, cruel and thankless labour, and slavery in the colonies helped to make Britain rich. Coalbrookdale may have been an extraordinary place but it was by no means perfect.

A history that tells only of significant events and characters says little of the millions of people who lived more humbly. Even the vivid writings of geniuses such as Austen, Dickens and Trollope, though sometimes quasi-biographical, are but accounts of fictional characters. The Coalbrookdale Doctors and others in this story were real individuals who lived in a society that arguably changed more radically than in any society before or since. For doctors such as Benjamin and William, and especially for Edward and Benjamin junior, it was a time to set aside old assumptions about health and disease and adopt the innovations that began to make medicine effective. They lived through the years in which the modern world was conceived.

Chapter 2

Benjamin in Coalbrookdale: Surgeon Apothecary

Today the view from the top of the Coalbrookdale is much as Benjamin would have seen it two hundred years ago. The woods are still there, and scattered within them are the ironmasters' fine houses and the terraces and cottages of the forge and foundry workers. A railway viaduct now follows the downward curve of the land. It crosses the Upper Furnace Pool which supplied the great water wheel that blasted air into the furnace, and towers over the place once filled with foundries and forges. Standing by the Nineteenth-Century church at the top of the Dale one can imagine the sylvan peace that prevailed here before its fiery industry arose. The smoke, the noise and clamour that once told of labour and commerce have gone, replaced by a weather-beaten tranquillity that scarcely conceals its ancient history. Just over the brow of the hill to the north the land, where once were innumerable mine-workings and mounds of waste, is now covered by the housing estates of Telford New Town though the Dale itself has been spared.

By the mid-Eighteenth Century, about 4,500 people in some nine hundred families lived in the Parish of Madeley. In the Sixteenth Century iron ore was being extracted as well as coal, though the small-scale bloomeries which had been worked there gave way to the bigger, more productive brick-built furnaces like those already in use at nearby Shifnal.[13]

Benjamin Wright came to set up his business as apothecary in

---

13 Shaw, S. 'Shifnal Ironworks Accounts, 1583-90', in *Shropshire Historical Documents, A Miscellany,* Shropshire Records Series, Vol 4, Centre for Local History, University of Keele, 2000, p 1.

Coalbrookdale in 1775. Originally apothecaries formed a section of the grocery trade that specialised in the increasing number of imported spices and plants that could be used in medicines. Strictly speaking, only physicians could diagnose illness but, because there were so few of them, especially in provincial counties like Shropshire, apothecaries began to do so themselves and then provide the necessary medicine. They therefore dissociated themselves from the grocers but continued to sell some of their customary goods such as tea, toiletries and household commodities, so their status remained that of shopkeepers and tradesmen. The growing population of the Dale must have provided plenty of work for an apothecary: the imperfect sanitary conditions encouraged infections and epidemics; working in the mines and at the furnaces exposed the labourers to accidents or even death; the rising birth rate encouraged a new trend for surgeons to attend women in childbirth — the so-called 'man-midwifery'. Coalbrookdale offered a good commercial opportunity for Benjamin Wright because, when he arrived, there was no one else in the area to compete with him, although two other apothecaries arrived in Madeley in the 1770s and were joined by another a few years later.

Effective medicines were few, though all manner of concoctions were prescribed and sold with a confidence that promised results that could rarely be delivered. Extracts of home-grown willow bark, the original source of aspirin, and of imported Cinchona or 'Peruvian bark', were quite effective for relieving the symptoms of fevers and agues, including malaria which was then common in some parts of Britain. Imported plant-based medicines such as ginger, peppermint and Turkish rhubarb were prescribed for the all-too-common indigestion, vomiting and diarrhoea. Patients with dropsy might be given costly imported medicines such as scammony, gamboge or jalap, until the Birmingham physician William Withering (who was born in Wellington, Shropshire) discovered that digitalis, from foxglove leaf, was more effective. The only worthwhile medicine to relieve severe pain was opium, either as laudanum (a tincture, or alcoholic extract) or paregoric (a tincture with camphor). Other commonly used medicines came from plants such as saffron from Italy and Spain, cinnamon from Sri Lanka and lobelia from North America, as well as home-grown colchicum, camomile and dandelion among many others. Salts of mercury, antimony and lead were favoured by physicians but their poisonous properties could be more dangerous than the diseases they were supposed to cure.

Apothecaries made their money by the sale of medicines, because according to the rules laid down by physicians to protect their own incomes, they were not allowed to charge for visiting or advising on the illness. They sold their medicines from shops but would also visit patients who were unable to leave their homes. The shops would have been simple affairs, usually a part of their dwelling-house but accessible to the public by a street door. Old prints of such shops in wealthy places show finely appointed rooms but Benjamin's would have been much less ornate: a counter to serve customers, a work-bench with the necessary pestle and mortar, scales and apparatus for distilling liquids or making pills, and shelves and drawers to hold the stock ingredients. There would have been space for the customers to wait their turn and a few chairs for the lame or weak to rest upon. The floor would be covered in surgical litter and other rubbish and in sawdust to help to clear out the mud from customers' boots.

Though he called himself a surgeon as well as apothecary, Benjamin would not have done any major operations, which were only undertaken in extreme cases. His surgical repertoire was the treatment of injuries, fractures and abscesses, and various procedures dictated by contemporary thinking on the cause of disease, for example the treatment of fevers by cupping, blistering or scarifying.[14] For centuries

---

14 Blistering: the application of irritants to the skin to cause effusion of fluid and blood. In Cupping, the same result was achieved by applying a heated glass cup which sucked fluid from the skin as it cooled. Scarifying was scratching the skin with a multi-bladed knife to draw blood.

it was supposed that illnesses were caused by imbalance of the four bodily humours — blood, phlegm and yellow or black bile — and that cure depended on reducing whichever humour was in excess. Thus all manner of symptoms were treated by removing 'bad blood' by cupping, blistering or the application of up to a dozen leeches, slug-like creatures that hook painlessly onto skin and suck blood until their hunger has been assuaged. If those did not work, a vein was cut open and blood allowed to flow into a measuring-vessel, a process called 'breathing a vein'. Sometimes so much blood was taken in this way that the patient fainted, and if it was done repeatedly could even cause anaemia.

Making sense of symptoms was a problem even for a university-educated physician because the workings of the body and the nature of disease were scarcely understood. Diagnosis was based on the patient's symptoms and very little physical examination was ever undertaken. Treatment was therefore empirical, that is it depended on what seemed to work according to the conventions of the time, and was based on the beliefs of eminent doctors rather than the well-considered evidence that would be required today. Anyone could 'invent' a medicine and promote it with persuasive advertising so the market was awash with hundreds of proprietary remedies such as 'Dr' Solomon's Balm of Gilead, Daffy's Elixir and Dr Radcliffe's drops to name but a few. Though Radcliffe was an eminent physician, neither Solomon nor Daffy had any medical training. These popular cures would have been available in many places including apothecaries' shops where they often competed with the proprietor's own '*nostrum*', meaning 'our own preparation'. But we should not dismiss the doctors of Benjamin's time as useless because there is more to medicine than medicines: in times of illness and stress the advice and compassion of experienced carers does much to support and comfort the sufferer. A trusted and knowledgeable person would have been a valuable member of a community such as Coalbrookdale. Benjamin would have shared the anxieties of parents when their children were ill.

He would have been a source of comfort to husbands and wives whose loved-ones were in danger from smallpox or pneumonia, and a support to relatives mourning a death. If the doctors of the time preserved a certain mystique in their methods, they did so to bolster their self-esteem and to reassure their patients as well as to obscure their forgivable ignorance.

Until the Eighteenth Century the care of women in childbirth had traditionally been undertaken by other women who would only turn to a surgeon for help if the birth was seriously complicated or the mother's condition was desperate. Many midwives accumulated considerable skill and competence, but without a clear understanding of its processes and complications, childbirth can be dangerous and, regrettably, not all midwives at this time were well-informed or competent. In an open market for medical attention, this field began to arouse the interest of surgeons such as John Knyveton in London who developed a prosperous man-midwifery practice.[15] Benjamin Wright certainly practised midwifery since his name appears as witness to the births of the children of Abraham Darby III.[16] Deborah Darby (1754-1810) records that he attended the Darby household on other occasions, saying that he was the doctor 'always called by the family'.[17]

The expansion of apothecary-surgeons into midwifery increased their incomes but added responsibility and a heavy burden of work, as shown by the records of Thomas Higgins of the small town of Wem in Shropshire. He was a contemporary of Benjamin's who had a large

---

15 Gray, E., *Man-midwife, the diary of John Knyveton,* London, Robert Hale Limited, re-printed 1944.

16 Julie Wright, descendant of Benjamin Wright, personal communication, 2010.

17 Labouchere, R., *Deborah Darby of Coalbrookdale, 1754-1810,* William Session Ltd, York, 1993, p 30.

midwifery practice from 1780 to his death in 1803.[18] During those twenty-three years his practice area was more than twelve miles across and in it he attended over one thousand deliveries, an average of one a week. This was a considerable workload to be done at any hour of the day or night and in all weathers, when the only means of transport was on horseback over bad and unlit roads or near-impassable lanes. Higgins's midwifery account books record the names and ages of his patients, the time and outcome of the births, the sex of the baby and whether they were live or still births — all in Latin. In a sample of a hundred of his cases, there were eighty-seven live single births, three sets of live twins and ten stillbirths, so the outcomes were good by the standards of the time. He also recorded his fees, which were usually 10s 6d or 15 shillings, but might be as much as 1 guinea if the birth was complicated or the patient well-to-do. Unfortunately for him, the bills often remained unpaid for months or years. The average fee was just over 13 shillings, which would have added £30 to the gross takings of his shop of about £350 a year, a considerable bonus when a personal income of £200 a year was considered generous.

The only information about Benjamin's medical practice that survives is contained in three sheets of paper recording the names and addresses of a few patients, with brief notes about the medicines prescribed and the fees charged. They are undated but may be from about 1785-90.[19] When he attended Thomas Baugh of Madeley Wood, he charged 1s 6d for the medicine and the same for going to visit him, recorded as 'a journey', but according to the rules he could not charge for deciding what was wrong or what medicine should be advised. Thomas Whittington at Lawley Bank was charged 1s 6d for a bottle of '*Mist. Card. Saline*', (cardamom was a spice from Malabar in India,

---

18 Tomkins, A. *The registers of a provincial man-midwife, Thomas Higgins of Wem 1781-1803*, in Shropshire Historical Documents, a Miscellany, Shropshire Record Series, Centre for Local History, University of Keele, 2000.

19 Iron Bridge Museum Trust Library

used as a stimulant) and the same for the journey, but the medicine seems not to have cured the problem because Benjamin had to go again two weeks later. For John Tranter of Dale House Farm he prescribed terebinth, a kind of turpentine often mixed with liquorice and honey and intended as a diuretic. Tranter must have gone to the shop, because no charge was made for a journey. John Rose, perhaps the Mr Rose who managed the Coalport porcelain works, was given opium in the form of *Elixir Paregoric* and some ointment, probably for painful arthritis, at a cost of 1s 4d. The cheapest charges were sixpence for liniments or ointments, and the most costly was to Mr Baugh of Sutton who was charged two shillings for some James's Powders. This medicine was one of the most commonly prescribed treatments for fever and was often sold as a ready-made proprietary remedy. Its principal ingredient was antimony which was known to be poisonous even in quite small doses, but despite this was frequently prescribed by physicians and commonly used in proprietary medicines.

One attendance by Benjamin on the Darby household is recorded in these papers. He went to their house, next door to his own, because such important patients would not have been expected to mingle with the *hoi polloi* shuffling through the sawdust on the floor of the shop. He attended Mrs Darby (probably Deborah) and Miss Appleby for symptoms which were not recorded. He prescribed a chalybeate (iron-containing) powder and a gentian extract for Mrs Darby and an emetic mixture for Miss Appleby at a total cost of 5s 6d. On another occasion he prescribed a syrup and turpentine for Abraham Darby III at sixpence each, for an unspecified complaint. In the days before accurate diagnosis was usual, or even possible, it was important to record the prescription given so that if the symptoms were relieved but re-occurred the same medicine could be used again — or avoided if there was no improvement.

Other imported medicines which Benjamin might have used include cinnamon from India, nutmeg (Malaya), myrrh (Abyssinia), strychnine (East Indies) and pareira root (Brazil). But he may have been sparing with such expensive ingredients because he had to make a profit on his business and most of his patients were not rich. In this snapshot of Benjamin's work there is only one reference to midwifery, for attendance on an un-named woman. Although the labour must have been hers, the entry in the accounts refers to *Mr* M. Gilpin,[20] presumably her husband, whose second contribution to the lady's pregnancy was to pay the fee of one guinea — as much as Thomas Higgins ever charged. Unlike Higgins's meticulous records, Benjamin's do not say whether it was boy, a girl or both who brought joy to the Gilpin family.

One dramatic case treated by Benjamin is publicly acknowledged. He played a significant role in saving the life of a child. One day in 1786, two-and-a-half-year-old Thomas Turner wandered away from home and fell into one of the ponds supplying the waterwheels that powered the machinery. Benjamin was hastily called to the scene even though Thomas was thought to have been in the water for half an hour and witnesses believed he was already dead.[21] Fortunately Benjamin knew the life-saving methods of the Royal Humane Society, formed only twelve years earlier by a group of doctors alarmed at the frequent and needless loss of life by drowning. In London, where there had been over 120 such deaths in one year, there was much concern because some victims had been pronounced dead while still capable of recovery.[22] The techniques devised by the Society were taught to local doctors throughout Britain, and Benjamin was one of twenty-seven

---

20 A Mr Mark Gilpin was clerk to the Coalbrookdale Company in 1794, personal communication from Sue Hemming, quoting Coalbrookdale Company archives.

21 Sue Hemming, personal communication with copies of correspondence from Benjamin Wright to the Royal Humane Society, 1786, and from the Society to an enquirer in 1905.

22 Royal Humane Society website, www.royalhumanesocety.org.uk, accessed 16 December 2012.

such 'Medical Assistants' in Shropshire.[23] Three-quarters of an hour after Thomas had been pulled from the pool there was still no sign of life but Benjamin persisted in his efforts to revive the boy using the methods of the Humane Society, including warming him with hot bricks. After a further hour the boy was '… so far recovered as to be able to speak' and the next day was 'perfectly restored'. As an incentive to promote life-saving skills, Medical Assistants could apply to the Royal Humane Society for a payment of four guineas for 'successfully bringing someone back to life'. Benjamin accordingly applied for his reward and, because such a long time had elapsed before Thomas recovered, the Society awarded him their Large Silver Medal for his persistence. He surely also earned the lasting gratitude of Thomas's parents who had been saved from the grief of losing their son.

Benjamin's activities were not only medical. As a prominent member of the community he was expected to contribute to the work of Madeley Parish Council. At this time local affairs were the responsibility of the parochial church councils whose members were elected by the more affluent parishioners. The parish was part of the established Anglican Church of course, so, strictly speaking, dissenters such as Roman Catholics, Jews and Quakers were not eligible for appointment to its councils. It is therefore remarkable that the rules were disregarded to allow admission of Benjamin Wright and Abraham Darby III who were non-conformists. Parish council members took responsibility in turn for various activities such as maintenance of the roads under a 'surveyor', the care of the poor under an 'overseer' and apprehension of offenders by a 'constable' (this was long before there was a police force). The minutes of Madeley Parish Council for the years 1780-94 show that for much of this time Benjamin was Overseer of the Poor, with responsibility for supporting those who were penniless

---

23 Advertisement, *Shrewsbury Chronicle,* 6 Sep 1777.

or too old or ill to earn a living.[24] This mostly involved distributing small doles of money to people in temporary difficulty or arranging admission of the destitute and homeless to the poor house, whose inmates he may also have attended as the parish doctor. Hannah Whale was allowed one shilling a week for a year and Widow Walton thirteen shillings to last until the following June, but Catherine Reynolds was given only sixpence a week. These women were entitled to this support because they had always lived in the parish but migrants from elsewhere were sent back to their home authority. Parishes could not afford to support outsiders because there was no government subsidy and all funds were raised locally and, consequently, the question of who should pay the cost of returning them to their own parishes was often a matter of dispute. As Overseer of the Poor Benjamin would have been involved in many such cases. When Madeley councillors sent Edward Stephenson back to Kington, fifty miles away in Herefordshire, at a cost £5 3s including £3 for hiring a horse, they applied to Kington for reimbursement of their expenses. The claim for the horse was rejected as illegal, but one guinea towards it was offered. Madeley reluctantly accepted the compromise and Benjamin put his signature to the relevant minute under those of several other council members.

In the days before there was a bank on every high street, money dealings could be arranged by those who handled cash such as apothecaries and other trades-people. Among Benjamin's few surviving papers there are four pages recording the names of people between whom money passed that was clearly not part of his medical business.

---

24 SA, 2280/6/95, Minutes of Madeley parish council, 1780-94.

Most of these are for relatively small amounts of between five and ten pounds, some of which, not being round figures, may have been payments for goods or services rather than loans or ready cash. There are many for much larger sums of £70 or £100, however, and two of over £200 — huge amounts at the time which would have kept a household in considerable comfort for a year.[25] The names of many of the parties to such deals are of locally eminent people, such as James Rathbone, Thomas Sutton, R. Guest and Abraham Darby III. Was Benjamin Wright the unofficial banker for Madeley or merely the trusted recorder and witness of such transactions? Or was he hoping to derive additional income by loans and investments in the way that others did so successfully, such as his colleague Dr Robert Darwin the eminent physician of Shrewsbury.[26] There are some sixty entries in these documents, all dated between 1786 and 1788 and, if this system extended over a longer period of years, Benjamin may have facilitated two hundred or more such transactions. A selection of the entries is shown in Table 2.1.

Other documents seem to show a list of bills drawn by named individuals upon others and payable to a third party, which are presumably borrowings or debts. Neither the sums involved nor the dates of the transactions are recorded. Each one has a serial number, the extant ones running from number 1,631 to 1,700, suggesting that there were up to two thousand or more of these transactions (Table 2.2 Overleaf). This appears to be a record of loans between the parties involved in which Benjamin was a broker.

Novels of the day frequently mention this system of borrowing, often describing the dire consequences if payment failed, but the

---

25 A sum of £100 in 1790 is equivalent to about £10,000 today, whereas an income of the same figure would be like one of £130,000, based on average earnings, www.measuringworth.com, accessed 22 Dec. 2012.

26 Pattison, A. *The Darwins of Shrewsbury*, The History Press, Stroud, Gloucestershire, 2009, p.72.

Table 2.1

A selection of financial transactions recorded by Benjamin Wright

Date	Time	Received of	Paid to	£	s	d
7 Nov 88	On Demand	R. Guest	A. Darby	5	5	-
11 May 87	Demand	Roger Cook	Ab. Darby	5	5	-
1 Jul 88	2 Mos	Thos Sutton	Ja^s Wright	20	-	-
18 Jul 88	2 Mos	Wm Goodman	James Wright	81	7	6
16 Aug 88	2 months	Ja^s Rathbone	John Horton	200	-	-
13 Sept 88	45 days	J. Rathbone	Fuller and Co	231	5	8

Table 2.2

A selection from the list of Bills drawn between three parties, as recorded by Benjamin Wright

Number	Drawn by	On whom Drawn	Payable unto
1642	Samuel Southall	Sam¹ & Thos Nicholson	John Atkinson
1658	John Wilkinson	Smith Wright & Gray	C. Guest
1659	Thos Wright Jun, Bristol	Goodshore Wigan & Co	Warron Jane
1676	Richard Reynolds	Smith Wright & Gray	John Onions
1673	Kinnersley and Co	Chas Reynolds	The Bearer

extent of Benjamin's exposure in such risks is not clear. Such large sums are unlikely to have accumulated solely from his medical business in which his charges were counted in shillings and pence, not tens and hundreds of pounds. It may be that he had inherited some capital from his father's farm and he was putting it to good use in this way. Whatever the correct interpretation, these documents suggest that this system of money lending and transfer was commonplace in the community of Coalbrookdale and that Benjamin Wright was a trusted and honourable intermediary in it.

So much for Benjamin's business responsibilities, but what of his personal life? In 1770, within two years of his marriage to Frances, their first baby, Mary, was born. Then, in 1771, came their second daughter, Elizabeth, who was to play an important role in this story as the wife of the second doctor of Coalbrookdale and the mother of his successors. In due course Benjamin and Frances had eight children and, though one of them died young, those who grew up and married presented their parents with fifty-six grandchildren.

In the course of the next twenty years Benjamin built a successful medical business, as shown by his attendance on the Darbys and other prominent people in the Dale, and was a leading member of the community involved in local affairs. By the 1790s he seems to have accumulated substantial financial resources or at least had access to them whether through Frances, by inheritance or through his own financial activities and business. In May 1791, when he was forty-six years of age, he leased land from Lord Craven, one of the principal landowners in the increasingly industrialized area of east Shropshire.[27] Benjamin took a sixty-three-year lease on nineteen acres in the parish of Little Dawley, on which there were 'several closes and enclosed grounds' with such names as 'The Garden of Dale Piece' and 'Bucknall's Rough'. Although this land was in the neighbouring parish it was only a few

---

27 SA, 1987/2/1, Copy Lease between Rt. Hon. William Lord Craven and Benjamin Wright.

hundred yards from Rosehill, the house where Benjamin had been living for years. The lease was subject to certain reservations, among which Lord Craven retained access to the Upper Furnace Pool and the use of the 'rail way'[28] which crossed the land from Coalbrookdale to the iron works at Horse Hay, though Benjamin was to be compensated for any damage caused by such use. Lord Craven also reserved for himself the timber on the land and any 'lops, tops and shreds' from it which were an important source of charcoal for the furnaces and forges. The most valuable reservations, however, were the coal, iron and limestone that lay below the surface. And, for good measure, his lordship retained the right of 'all manner of Hawking, Hunting, Coursing, Shooting, Fishing and Sporting': the pleasures and pastimes of the aristocracy were not to be discarded lightly.

The agreement specified that within three years Benjamin would 'expend the sum of £600 at least in erecting ... a good substantial messuage[29] or tenement and out offices ... on some convenient part of the premises'. By this time he had been the doctor in Coalbrookdale for more than twenty years, and if his medical and non-medical interests were as profitable as it seems, his prospects were good. He was a family man with seven living children and, though he already rented a comfortable house at Rosehill, he wished to have property of his own appropriate to his position. Like many prosperous people of his time he was nurturing the ambition to live as a gentleman, to educate his sons well and move in the right circles for his daughters to find husbands. Building a fine new house compatible with his status in the community would help to achieve all this but at the considerable

---

28 This was actually a iron plate way on which wagons ran, rather than a modern 'railway'

29 Messuage: a portion of land occupied, or intended to be occupied, as the site for a dwelling house and its appurtenances: in later use, a dwelling house together with its outbuildings and the adjacent land assigned to its use. Oxford English Dictionary, on-line edition accessed 13 Dec 2012.

cost of '£600 *at least*'. On this land Benjamin built Green Bank Farm, so called because of its situation in the green fields on the bank of the Upper Furnace Pool which had been made by damming the Loamhole Brook that drains the valley. Surrounded by its nineteen acres, it faced the open space of the pool across which could be seen his former home of Rosehill with a fine view of the wooded slopes of the lower Dale if the less attractive furnaces and forges were disregarded.

Alas, Benjamin did not enjoy the rewards of his prosperity for long. Although his calling was to tend the sick, he was no more immune to disease and mortality than his neighbours and patients. On 3 January 1794, Rebecca Darby noted in her diary that ...'a neighbour and acquaintance has for some weeks laboured under great disposition, I mean Benjamin Wright. He was the surgeon who attended the births of some of the Darby children and well-known to them all'.[30] Benjamin's 'disposition' was indeed 'great', for he died on 15th February aged only 49 years, and was buried in the Quaker burial ground eight days later.[31]

Though always unexpected, death at this early age was not unusual. In Chadwick's famous report in the late 1830s, the average age at death of professional people was said to be between forty and fifty years depending on the locality.[32] In Coalbrookdale there had been untimely deaths in the Darby family, too: Abraham I was thirty-nine when he died, Abraham II was fifty-two, Abraham III was thirty-nine and Samuel was forty-four. This despite the fact that people in uncrowded country districts lived, on average, ten years longer than those in densely populated and polluted cities and professional people several years more than their labouring neighbours. Despite these low average ages at death, many people continued into their eighties or

---

30 From *Letters of Rebecca Darby,* 3 January 1794, p 252.

31 National Archives, RG 6/457, 00084, Instruction to Thomas Roberts, Grave Maker.

32 Chadwick, E., *The Sanitary Condition of the Labouring Population of Great Britain, 1842.* Flinn, M.W., (ed.), Edinburgh University Press, 1965, 200.

nineties, so Benjamin's death must be considered premature even by the standards of two hundred years ago. What could have caused such an untimely death? Rebecca Darby noted in early January that Benjamin had been ill for 'some weeks' after which he lived another month, so his illness was a prolonged one. According to Chadwick, in 1838 there were more than 1,700 deaths in Shropshire from one of six infectious diseases, and although admittedly this was more than forty years after Benjamin died it indicates a likely situation in the 1790s. Over half of these deaths were due to tuberculosis, recorded as 'consumption', and more than a hundred each to measles and scarlet fever. There were 150 deaths from smallpox and 240 from pneumonia, both of which would probably have been shorter illnesses than the three months or more that Benjamin suffered. A likely cause of Benjamin's death is typhus, a lingering disease of fever, debility and mental confusion which at that time was fatal in about one case in ten — surely a 'great disposition'. Because typhus is carried by body lice it is prevalent where hygiene is bad, so Benjamin's work in labourer's cottages and as Overseer of the Poor and doctor in the Poor House would have exposed him to the risk of infection.

Whatever the cause of Benjamin's untimely death, he left a grieving widow and a family of teenage children, and the community lost its doctor. The vacancy for an apothecary-surgeon in Coalbrookdale was soon filled by the twenty-two year old William Edwards who married Benjamin's daughter Elizabeth. Benjamin's business and his family lived on into the next century.

Chapter 3
William

Benjamin and Frances's oldest child, Mary, was already twenty-four years old when her father died but Ann, the youngest, was not yet eight. Their first son James died young so the oldest surviving boy was Peter, who was old enough in 1794 to be apprenticed to his father but too young to have qualified and too inexperienced to take on the business. His occupations have been described as farmer, agent and gentleman and occasionally he was referred to as 'Surgeon Wright', though his name does not appear in any medical directory. Benjamin's will, dated 13th February 1794, only two days before he died, provides that all his property be used to support his widow Frances and to bring up and educate their seven surviving children. It does not mention succession to the business.

The next documented event in this part of the story is the marriage of Elizabeth, Benjamin and Frances's second child, to William Edwards, apothecary and surgeon. He had taken over the business at some point, though it is unclear whether he came while Benjamin was alive, or at some later time. The wedding took place on 8th February 1796 at Dawley Magna church, in the parish in which the Wright family's new home, Green Bank, is situated. William and Elizabeth moved into Rose Hill, now 43 Darby Road, where William carried on the business, while Frances and her other children remained at Green Bank.

William was the younger son of Richard Edwards and his wife Mary (née Fuller) who had a small estate at Water Newton in Cambridgeshire. His date of birth is uncertain though his baptism is recorded as 25th June 1775 so he was only about twenty-one or twenty-two years of age when he married Elizabeth. There were strong family connections with this part of Shropshire. William's paternal grandfather, Edward, was born in Broseley and married Katherine (née Hinckesman) from Neen Savage, not far from Broseley, where they lived before buying the Cambridgeshire property. William's older brother Richard who was a graduate of St John's College, Cambridge, and became a curate at Wilton in Wiltshire was living in Shrewsbury in 1805 but moved from there to London. Although William did not go to university he received a classical education, as observations in subsequent letters confirm. Where he had his early education is unknown, but it may have been privately as a pupil of a local clergymen, like many boys who entered the medical profession as apothecaries or surgeons at this time.[33] Others such as Erasmus and Charles Darwin, sons of the Shrewsbury physician Robert Darwin, went to their local grammar school where the syllabus was confined to the classics and 'a little geography and history' with no mathematics or science at all.[34]

It is therefore a matter of speculation as to how William came to take over Benjamin's medical business and how he met his future wife Elizabeth. It is reasonable to suppose that family relationships had secured for him an apprenticeship to an apothecary in their old home town of Broseley, which would have put him in a favourable position when the vacancy in Coalbrookdale occurred. In Broseley he may have met Benjamin Wright's father-in-law John Guest, ironmaster and acquaintance of the Darbys, and could have been engaged by Benjamin's executors, his brother Peter and brother-in-law Charles Guest of Broseley, to run the business as *locum tenens,* and thus to meet Elizabeth. It may have been agreed that he would become an assistant to Benjamin when he completed his apprenticeship, which was forestalled by Benjamin's early death. William and Elizabeth might even have been teenage sweethearts. The details of their romance and his entry to the business are therefore left to the reader's imagination.

---

33 Loudon, I., *Medical Care and the General Practitioner, 1750-1850.* Oxford, The Clarendon Press, 1986, pp 36-7.

34 Darwin, C., *Autobiographies,* London, Penguin Classics, 1986.

However that may be, by 1796 William had become the second Coalbrookdale doctor, and lived at Rose Hill where he and Elizabeth brought up their family of eight children — a fair share of Benjamin and Frances Wright's fifty-six grandchildren.

The business of apothecary being learned by apprenticeship, Benjamin and William would have been apprenticed to a master apothecary for five to seven years for a premium of £200-300, probably paid by their fathers. The master undertook to teach his pupil the knowledge and skills of the trade and provide food and lodging but not clothing while the pupil undertook to study diligently and help with the business. The apprentice had to behave himself properly: specifically to 'keep the master's secrets' and 'do no damage'; to refrain from playing at cards, gambling or visiting taverns and playhouses; to avoid fornication and not be married.[35] A typical advertisement for a 'Medical Apprentice' sought a 'youth of 15 or 16', for whom the advertiser ensured that:—

> Every part of his profession (and its connection with comparative anatomy) [will be] carefully pointed out, and his reading, morals and domestic comforts, will be particularly attended to.

The advertisement emphasises the educational opportunities but, once the premium had been paid, the young men were ripe for exploitation. At best a good master would fulfil his obligations but the phrase 'every part of his profession' included sweeping the shop and washing the bottles, and 'reading' might imply no more than learning the doggerel Latin in which prescriptions were written. By the time William started his training, however, apprenticeship alone was not enough, as it had been in Benjamin's day. By the end

---

35 SA, M1268/1, William Masefield's apprenticeship indenture to Henry Somerville, 1815.

of the Eighteenth Century apothecaries were not only dispensers of medicines but were actually practising medicine and surgery, both in their shops (which thus became known as 'surgeries') and by visiting patients in their homes. Master apothecaries could not provide facilities for the anatomical dissection and surgical experience now required to meet rising educational standards. Students began to spend some months in London attending lectures and 'walking the wards' of the hospitals to improve their theoretical knowledge and practical skills. In William's time medical schools did not exist in London but many surgeons gave courses of lectures and provided facilities for dissection, a side-line which increased their incomes and brought them to greater prominence with the public. But living in London was expensive and money had to be found for lecture fees, books and instruments. William's older brother Richard had been to university but their father seems to have found the cost of William's study in London on top of his apprenticeship premium rather beyond his means. Fortunately a bachelor uncle, Captain Edward Edwards RN (of whom we will hear more later) came to the rescue by lending William £200 for his London studies. William repaid the loan in due course. Had he failed to do so, he would have forfeited an inheritance of £500 from his maternal grandmother, Ann Hewison of Godmanchester, the mother of his avuncular benefactor.[36] By his early twenties William had had five years of medical education and was ready to set up in business. As there was no formal test of competence, William had only to satisfy his master that he was capable of working as an apothecary-surgeon.

At this time the private medical schools in London attracted students from all over the country. Nowhere else in England could students of surgery learn from the best teachers and get such good experience as in the many hospitals of the capital. The smaller provincial infirmaries offered facilities for study and practice but experience was

---

36 National Archives, X 806/21, The will of Anne Hewison of Godmanchester, 16 July 1794.

limited. The system of training by apprenticeship supplemented by study in London was the start of many students' rise to fame. For example, Dr John Langdon Down MD, the first to describe Down's syndrome, was the son of an apothecary in Torpoint in Devon who studied in this way and eventually settled in London with a large practice.[37] William Marsden, founder of both the Royal Free and the Royal Marsden hospitals, moved from Sheffield to London to be an apothecary's apprentice and medical student and eventually took his MD.[38] Sir James Paget, physician to St Bartholomew's Hospital and remembered for 'Paget's Disease' of bone, began as an apprentice in Great Yarmouth.[39] Most influential of all, perhaps, was Thomas Wakley who was apprenticed to an apothecary in Taunton. He later founded *The Lancet*, an incisively radical journal, and as a Member of Parliament advocated many reforms of the medical profession and its autocratic institutions.[40]

This system of local experience supplemented by study in London may seem inadequate compared with the ten or more years of study now required but it was the standard procedure for many aspiring young men of the time. London was not alone, however, because students could also go to Edinburgh or Glasgow, where the courses were better structured, and some even went to European schools. The Royal College of Physicians and the Company of Surgeons (later renamed the Royal College of Surgeons) controlled the professions in London and did not recognise these 'foreign' schools. This policy was intended to thwart unqualified quacks and charlatans competing with their members but

---

37 Ward, Conor, *Dr John Langdon Down and Normansfield,* London, Langdon Down Centre Trust, undated.

38 Sandwith, F., *Surgeon Compassionate, the story of Willaim Marsden,* Peter Davies, 1960.

39 Newman, C., The Evolution of Medical Education in the Nineteenth Century, Oxford University Press, 1957, p 38.

40 Oxford DNB, on-line edition, Thomas Wakley, accessed 25 Jun 2013.

it also prevented well-educated Scottish or European graduates from setting up practice in London. These properly qualified doctors were prosecuted for infringing rules designed for a different purpose.

William's case records and account books have not survived so we must illustrate the nature of his work from extant records of his contemporaries. One such is William Pulsford of Wells in Somerset, only slightly earlier.[41] Nearly one third of Pulsford's recorded cases were fractures or other injuries, often caused by falling from or being kicked by horses or by tumbling off ladders or trees. In an area like Coalbrookdale, where men worked with burning coal and molten metal, handled heavy objects or drove wagons loaded with ore and limestone, injuries such as burns, fractures and contusions must have been frequent. Another contemporary of William's, William Thackrah of Leeds, studied the effect on the workers of conditions in various industries, and produced what is probably the first study of occupational health.[42] He noticed that the respiration of men working in 'sulphurous and smoky departments' was often affected, but he believed that, though many men were pallid and thin, this was rarely due to consumption. He observed that although iron-founders, of whom there were many at Coalbrookdale, were exposed to great heat, sweated profusely and drank huge amounts of beer this 'did not produce sensible or immediate disorder'. One man actually admitted to drinking 'six or seven *quarts* a day' — probably of very low-alcohol 'small beer'. On the other hand, Thakrah noted that men who were exposed to dust, especially from 'draw-filing' which produced very small particles, showed signs of respiratory disease when quite young, and few such men were still fit for employment over the age of fifty. William dealt with the same kind of problems in Coalbrookdale as Thakrah did in Leeds, as he reported to the Manchester physician Thomas Percival:

---

41 Loudon, I., *Medical Care and the General Practitioner, 1750-1850.*

42 Meiklejohn, A., *The Life, Work and Times of Charles Turner Thackrah, 1795-1883*, London, E. & S. Livingstone, 1957, pp 97-8 and 151-2.

> I have never observed that asthmas [*sic*] and other pulmonary affections are more frequent in the Dale than elsewhere, but rather to the contrary. Old colliers and such as work in iron, stone-mines and lime rocks are very subject, in the decline of life, to coughs and shortness of breath, especially hard drinkers; but in other respects the inhabitants are remarkably healthy ... the smoke arising from coal and iron not being so prejudicial as from copper works in Cornwall and other parts. Such colliers and miners as are troubled with coughs always ascribe it to the dust arising in getting the mineral, and the smoke in the burning of lime, for which they take frequent emetics and purges.[43]

William was powerless to prevent these early cases of pneumoconiosis and his emetics and purges would do little to cure the disease.

Another large part of Pulsford's work, and presumably William's, was treating infections such as smallpox, typhus, venereal diseases, scarlet fever and erysipelas.[44] The next most common problems were local infections such as boils and abscesses, and ulcerated legs which were considered to be so incurable that such patients were excluded from hospitals like the Salop Infirmary. Though no medicine could cure these conditions in William's time it was his duty to help his patients through their ordeals. The records of another contemporary, Dr Loxham in Lancashire, also show that half of his cases were fevers, infectious diseases, lacerations and fractures.[45] Loxham had a large obstetric practice, as did William,

---

43 Percival, Thomas, *Medical Ethics,* London, 1803, Note XIX, Correspondence with William Edwards of Coalbrookdale, pp 234-237.

44 Erysipelas is caused by the same germ as scarlet fever and produces large red eruptions on the skin. It is highly infectious and in William's time it was often fatal.

45 King, S., *A Fylde Country Practice,* Centre for North-West Regional Studies, University of Lancaster, 2001, p 14.

so many of his cases were connected with childbirth and 'female complaints'. Cancer, which is now so common, was not recorded by Pulsford in three hundred cases but Loxham noted nine 'tumours', though whether they were malignant is uncertain and only those which could be seen, as in the breast or skin, could be diagnosed with any certainty. Pulsford made no mention of stroke or heart attack. Both recorded all kinds of minor troubles: pains in the limbs, sore eyes, piles, hernia, toothache, skin disease, 'the itch' (scabies) and many more. William's case load was probably similar. As mentioned earlier, apothecary surgeons were beginning to practise midwifery and William certainly did so, as his letters to his son Edward in the 1820s show. What proportion of his time was spent on this work is unknown, but in a place to which young people came to find work there was probably a high demand.

Partnership with colleagues was unusual in William's time, but it was common to employ an assistant or take an apprentice, as William did by employing Edward when he was old enough. He was therefore always at the beck and call of patients but without the conveniences of telephone and motor-car and certainly without modern diagnostic methods or support from specialists or hospitals. Patients who could walk would have been seen in the shop, but for housebound or bedridden patients he would have had to travel miles on horse-back to outlying farms or cottages, leaving the shop in charge of the apprentice. Emergencies and childbirth could demand his attention at any hour of the day or night and in all weathers.

A mid-Nineteenth Century author rather patronisingly described the country doctors of William's time as being rough in manners and limited in knowledge and skill, but mentioned two men of rather more respectable nature.[46] One, un-named but locally well known:

---

46 Jeafferson, W., *A Book about Doctors,* publisher un-named, undated (c1850).

> ... always went on his rounds on horseback booted and spurred. The state of the roads rendered any other mode of travelling impracticable to men who had to ... make their way up bridle-paths and drifts and lanes, to secluded farmsteads and outlying villages.

Another became famous in medical history:

> He was dressed in a blue coat and yellow buttons, buckskins, well-polished jockey-boots with handsome silver spurs, and he carried a smart whip with a silver handle. His hair, after the fashion, was done up in a club, and he wore a broad-brimmed hat.

This was Edward Jenner who famously observed that the deadly disease of smallpox could be prevented by inoculation with the less dangerous cowpox, and thus pointed the way to the eradication of one of the most dreadful epidemic diseases that mankind has ever suffered from. It has been said of Jenner that he was 'the means of saving more lives than any other man'.[47, 48]

Letters to Edward from his family in later years speak of the fatigue that William endured as a result of this demanding work and the effect that it had on his health. Visiting a patient at Eaton Constantine or Little Wenlock would involve a ride of ten or twelve miles, and though doctor's mounts were said to be steady and reliable

---

47 Jeafferson, W., *A Book about Doctors,* attributing the remark to Rowland Hill (1744-1833), a fervent non-conformist preacher and advocate of smallpox vaccination. This Rowland Hill was the sixth son of the wealthy Sir Rowland Hill of Hawkstone Park, Shropshire (but *not* the inventor of penny postage).

48 The introduction of vaccination over the next two decades was controversial. Though potentially dangerous it was one of very few advances in disease prevention in this period. Whether William used it is unknown.

they were not swift. The roads, even the main ones or turnpikes, were in bad repair and full of pot-holes, and some by-ways and bridle paths could be almost impassable.[49] Flood and rain that could penetrate even a broad-brimmed hat and heavy woollen cloak, and an hour's journey on horseback on a frosty night could be a demanding experience. The exhausted horse would be as badly affected as its rider. In 1814 William wrote to Edward, then in London, saying: 'My old horse is lame, and I am fearful he has seen his best days, he is like me [and] will not last for ever'.[50] In the same letter he regrets that he has 'hardly been at Church all Winter because the weather and business prevent me'. This was the year after Napoleon was frozen out of Russia. The strain of these journeys was already telling and William was only forty years old.

Elizabeth's letters to Edward mention some of William's patients and the problems he was dealing with:[51]

> Mrs J. Richards has been poorly since her last confinement she is getting better her mother sais she makes herself uneasy on account of her Husband coming home tipsy every night cou'd you have thought of such a thing. [*original spelling*].

> Francis's wife was oblig[d] to send for your father [for her confinement] the other night the doctor did not arrive in time.

---

49   Plymley, J., *General View of the Agriculture of Shropshire,* London, The Board of Agriculture, 1802, p 273.

50   Letter 2, 1987/56/15, William to Edward, 22 Feb 1814.

51   Letter 7, 1987/56/17, Elizabeth to Edward, 1 Jan 1822.

> Ralph Williams has met with a bad accident at the H[orse] Hay works his hand was dreadfully torn with a wheel he now comes down to have it dressed the smell is so offensive we can hardly bear the house when he comes your father will be poorly paid for such a job

She also mentions a touch of rivalry between the local doctors: Mrs Yate (her sister Fanny who married Timothy Yate) had been unwell but rather than consulting William she had 'employed Mr Bailey', another local doctor. Elizabeth said that 'Aunt Yate has been getting better' under her new doctor's care but that there was 'a little shyness amongst us'. Reading between the lines it seems that the doctor-patient relationship between William and his sister-in-law had failed. Another problem involved the Lightmoor Club, a self-help insurance system for the low-paid, where a dissatisfied patient named Baker had 'employed some old woman' who was nothing more than a quack. When the case went wrong Baker tried to blame William and have him sacked as the club doctor, but the allegation was not upheld and the patient transferred his allegiance to another doctor.[52] Perhaps William was relieved to lose a difficult patient.

In another letter Elizabeth mentioned William's difficulties with some of his midwifery cases:

> We are losing a great number [of mothers]. The cases are too numerous to mention, Mr Proctor sent for your father to a dangerous case last night, but the patient is likely to do well. Your father lost another labour on Tuesday.[53]

---

52 Letter 8, 1987/56/18, Elizabeth to Edward, 26 Jan 1822.

53 Letter 8, 1967/56/18, Elizabeth to Edward, 26 Jan 1822.

Though the risks of childbirth at this time were very high and death was not uncommon, such losses must have been distressing for all concerned. The mortality rate in Coalbrookdale is unknown but, since many women had ten or more children, the death of a mother in the very process of giving birth to another was a disaster for the family. The Salop Infirmary did not admit pregnant women but, even if there had been a lying-in hospital, mortality rates could be ten times higher than for home deliveries.[54] One of the most serious risks was from infection, usually by the same germ that causes scarlet fever and erysipelas, conditions that William was often called upon to treat. Though they did not realise it, doctors of William's time might infect women in childbirth with the germs of a fatal disease from another patient, perhaps a child with tonsillitis or a man with an inflamed leg.

Most patients would have been seen in the shop (or surgery, as we now say), but those who were socially superior or too ill to get there would have been seen at home. The houses of the well-to-do, such as the Darbys, the Baughs and the Gilpins, would be warm and clean but labouring families did not live so comfortably. In the mid-Eighteenth Century the Coalbrookdale Company built houses such as Carpenters Row and Nailers Row for their workers, and others may have been built by speculators, such as the 1740 Tea Kettle Row which still exists beside the doctors' house at Rose Hill. Others have been demolished, including Smokey Row (near the furnaces), School House Row and Charity Row, the latter built for the widows of company workmen. Although these houses were substantially built of brick with quarry-tile floors they were small — typically two rooms twelve feet square on the ground floor with two tiny bedrooms upstairs — and they were scarcely large enough for a family with several children. The furnishings were sparse: Mary Cadman had saved a few guineas when she married Thomas Cadman, enough to buy a bed, a few chairs,

---

54 Loudon, I., *The Tragedy of Childbed Fever,* Oxford University Press, 2000, p 60.

and some showy bits of furniture.[55] They may have added others later, but the wages, collected fortnightly on 'Reckoning Day', were usually spent on food and drink in the first few days, leaving little to spare for other comforts or possessions. There were exceptions of course: one clergyman complained that men's wages were so high they could afford luxuries and his wife said they had more money than her reverend husband; others said the men's money was wasted in ale houses or on such large Sunday dinners that they went hungry for the rest of the week.[56] Every company house had a larder and each row a communal brew-house and washhouse but water had to be carried from a nearby well that might easily be contaminated from the Row's 'long-drop' privies. If there was no well, water could be obtained from the polluted brook or, worse still, from the River Severn itself which was the final repository for the excreta of the people in riverside houses and the crews of innumerable boats. Hygienic it was not.

Those not fortunate enough to live in company houses might occupy one of the squatters' cottages, such as those at the top of the Dale in Holywell Lane between Little Dawley and Little Wenlock. In the 1820s there were twenty-five of them crowded together on roadside verges, with single-thickness brick walls and un-sawn roof timbers. One was only 12 x 11 feet square, few had as many as four rooms and the sanitation was of very doubtful quality. Sometimes even redundant engine houses, brick kilns and blast furnaces were adapted for housing. Four families lived in one converted engine house, and another had adapted a disused conical pottery kiln as a dwelling, which presented the difficulty of fixing a rectangular cupboard to a curving wall.[57] Such houses were no place to bring up children, and certainly not to give birth, possibly by candle light on a cold winter's night: no

---

55 Trinder, B., *The Industrial Revolution in Shropshire,* p 206.

56 Trinder, B., *The Industrial Revolution in Shropshire,* p 205.

57 Trinder, B., *The Industrial Revolution in Shropshire.* p 189.

wonder childbirth, measles and scarlet fever gave so much work to the doctors, and the undertakers too.

As well as the recurrent fear of French invasion, the disturbance to the national economy caused by the war had severe consequences, especially in Coalbrookdale. In the 1740s, the Coalbrookdale Company, under Abraham Darby II, did make cannons but, by the end of the century, the Quaker proprietors of the Coalbrookdale Company were pacifists and refused to make military hardware, although other foundries prospered from doing so. Yet even before the war the fortunes of the Dale were declining for other reasons. In 1795 the River Severn had flooded to an unusually high level, rising suddenly and unexpectedly to thirty inches more than the previous great flood of 1770. Though the high and stalwart Iron Bridge survived, the next bridge upstream at Buildwas 'blew up' and downstream two arches of the one at Bridgnorth were demolished by the torrent. Along the riverside at Coalbrookdale stocks of timber were washed away when a warehouse was swamped and several houses were so badly damaged that their occupants had to be taken to the workhouse for shelter.[58] Thomas Telford, then Surveyor to the county of Shropshire, recorded the season and its consequences as 'beyond all precedent':

> The storm of frost and Snow kept accumulating for two months, after which a very hasty Thaw caused a greater inundation than has ever been known in England. Much injury has been done by the various Rivers, and the Severn has not been behindhand; that and other Collateral Streams have demolished many Bridges in Shropshire.'[59]

---

58 Trinder, B., *The Industrial Revolution in Shropshire,* Chichester, Phillimore and Co, 1981, p 175.

59 Letter from Thomas Telford to Sir John Sinclair, 18 March 1795, quoted in Raistrick, R., *Dynasty of Ironfounders,* London, Longman Green and Co, 1953, p 205.

The flood was only one manifestation of the so-called 'little ice-age', a series of prolonged and severe winters in which the River Thames froze in London and 'Frost Fairs' were held on the foot-thick ice. Harvests in 1774 and 1782 had been bad, and that of 1795 was disastrous. Local sources of wheat had never been plentiful and, when harvests were bad, there was not enough to go round: even an extra slice or two of bread put a strain on household resources. It was said that the situation was compounded by a newly established habit of 'taking tea', an extra meal in late afternoon that required more bread. To supply this for all the nine hundred families in Madeley an extra 3,200 pounds of flour was needed which local sources could not supply, nor could it be obtained from elsewhere. Demand and prices rose as supply faltered, and it was reported that:

> Haggard hunger, despairing wretchedness and ignorant force were banded to trample down the safeguards of civil rights. Armed ruffians took the initiative to scramble for food'.[60]

The effect on the health of the population can only have added to the doctors' work because malnutrition led to scurvy, rickets and stunted growth.

Without a Welfare State and a National Health Service the plight of the poor could be desperate. In harsh winters, hunger could sometimes be mitigated if cottagers had a little land on which to keep a pig and grow vegetables but many of the cottages in the Dale lacked such advantage. Hunger posed such a threat that at one time it was reported that:

> Such is the temper of the people that there is not a day to lose if we are desirous to preserve the poor from

---

60 Randall, J., *History of Madeley*, p 74-5.

outrage, and most likely the country from plunder if not from blood.[61]

The employers tried to find a solution to the food crisis of 1795 because they feared that hungry workers would besiege or even destroy their offices and homes in violent demands for relief. A meeting of several employers at the Tontine Inn near the Iron Bridge was chaired by Richard Dearman of the Coalbrookdale Company and attended by George Forester, Cecil Forester and John Wilkinson and others. They agreed to buy 2,000 bushels of corn from Liverpool for distribution to the hungry families in the area.[62] But further bad harvests followed and the relief, though welcome, was only temporary. In 1796 employers from the surrounding area met again, but this time it was decided to buy rice rather than wheat which was scarce and costly. The Coalbrookdale Company subscribed £1,500 and other companies raised similar sums: £1,000 from Madeley Wood, £2,000 from Ketley Company for example. Rice was not the usual diet of people in the Dale and at first there was resentment and resistance to this dole, but at least it was food and it had to be accepted for want of an alternative.

Quite apart from the demands on the proprietors of the Coalbrookdale Company to pay for food, the financial crisis blocked the supply of credit. The stability of the Shrewsbury Bank was threatened by a run on banks that had started in Newcastle and had involved the Bank of England and others throughout the country.[63] The Coalbrookdale Company subscribed a large sum to support the Shrewsbury Bank which can only have added to the Company's problems and thus have affected the livelihoods of its employees.

---

61 Randall, J. *History of Madeley*, p 110.

62 A bushel is approximately 14.5 Kg. so 2000 bushels amounted to about 29 metric tons of corn.

63 Raistrick, A., *Dynasty of Ironfounders*, London, Longmans, Green and Co. 1953, p 221.

William succeeded Benjamin as the Coalbrookdale doctor in 1796, at the height of these crises, so it cannot have been an easy time for a twenty-two-year-old to enter practice. Because of the war and decline in the iron industry, conditions did not get easier for many years. Labouring people could pay for medical treatment if they were ill by subscribing a few pence a week to a local 'Sick Club' while they were well. This paid the doctors' fees but it was by no means a secure source of income for the doctor. In 1822, Elizabeth told Edward in a letter that the income from the sick clubs 'has rather fallen off this year'.[64] The Lightmoor Club was down by £1,5s, she wrote, because trade in the Dale was 'excessively flat' and 'the men do not get half [their usual] employment'. Unable to pay their subscriptions, the men could not claim if they were ill and so the doctor was not called and he received no payment. William told Edward that a club he had started 'had removed to Mrs Carter's at Dawley Green and [I] am afraid is rather on the Decline'.[65] More telling for William was the effect on his own costs and charges for the medicines he dispensed:

> Everything here is very dear, particularly Loaf Sugar, of which I am very sparing in the Shop. 20 oz of Oil of Almonds is worth 5s which makes Emulsions very dear for Club patients tho in great demand due to the inclemence of the Season. Eggs have been 3d each, Butchers meat 10d pd, it will be necessary that Physic [medicine] should rise as well as other things that the poor people cannot pay for as wages are very low'.[66]

---

64 Letter, 1987/56/17, Elizabeth to Edward, 1 Jan 1822.

65 Letter, 1987/56/15, William to Edward, 22 Feb 1814.

66 Letter, 1987/56/15, William to Edward, 22 Feb 1814.

They were hard times for the poor, for the doctor and his family, and even for the rich. Poverty threatens health and denies the resources for treatment; 'cutbacks' in health care are nothing new.

Trade was so bad in 1816-17 that the Coalbrookdale ironmasters imposed wage restrictions that provoked strikes. In Nottingham in 1811, changes to working practices in the textile factories caused unemployment and provoked the Luddite movement which tried to prevent change by destroying the new machines that employed fewer people. Similar violent challenges to authority occurred in Shropshire where the recession in the iron trade had reduced wages. Thus for more than twenty years William had to contend with the consequences of poverty and hardship among his patients in addition to accidents, midwifery and epidemics. During this time William and Elizabeth were financially constrained and William's letters often mention his financial difficulties.

William and Elizabeth had moved into Rose Hill soon after their marriage and it was there that Elizabeth gave birth to their eight children. From letters of later years it appears to have been a happy home. The first child to be born, in 1797, was their daughter Betsey, followed by their first son Edward in 1798. Richard was born in 1804 after an unusually long gap of six years (in which there may have been a miscarriage or still birth), and then Fanny (1807), Anna Maria (1810), William (1813), Mary (1815) and finally Benjamin in 1816. What could have been better? Elizabeth survived the risks of childbirth eight times, and her four boys and three of the four girls reached their teenage years. But tragedy shadowed their happiness: Mary died in infancy and Richard died aged seventeen in 1821. Young William was only fifteen and still at school when he too died. The causes of their deaths can only be guessed but they may have been due to infections such as scarlet fever or smallpox whose frequent and potent epidemics did not spare the young. So the male children were reduced to two boys, both of them destined to follow their father into his practice and maintain it until late in the nineteenth century. As for the girls, Betsey remained at home to keep house and support her brothers, while Fanny and Anna Maria sought other fortunes, though marriage was not for them either.

Some relief for William came when, in 1812 at the age of fourteen, Edward decided to follow his father's profession. He was a valuable assistant and promising student and soon developed a favourable reputation among the patients. At the age of fifteen Edward went to London to attend lectures and walk the wards of the city's hospitals, but such progress had been made in medical sciences that he needed more time than his father had taken twenty years earlier. The medical profession was being roused from its long slumber of unquestioning tradition to enter an era of science, education and re-organisation.

Chapter 4

Edward

As the Nineteenth Century progressed, the people of Coalbrookdale entered a period of mixed fortunes. William had plenty of work but his bills often remained unpaid and money was short. Food supplies in the Dale improved but winters were severe. Although there were thirty blast furnaces making fifty thousand tons of cast iron,[67] the industry remained in recession.

Despite continuing difficulties, under the leadership of Richard Reynolds the Coalbrookdale Company enjoyed a period of innovation and technical development. For decades the company had been making cylinders for steam engines to meet the rising demand for power, and there were at least 180 'fire-engines' in the area lifting 250,000 tons of coal a year and pumping water from the mines.[68] More efficient engines had been made possible by Wilkinson's new boring machines for making cylinders.[69] Meanwhile, the wooden plate-ways, along which horses hauled loaded carts, were replaced by more durable iron rails, also made in the Dale. And, in 1801, the Cornishman Richard Trevithick had the bright idea of creating an engine-on-wheels that he put into practice on a road at Camborne in Cornwall, though it was destroyed during trials.[70] The following year he worked with the Coalbrookdale Company to build a mobile, high-pressure steam

---

67 SA 1987/64/6.

68 Plymley, J., *General View of the Agriculture of Shropshire,* London, The Board of Agriculture, 1802, p 340

69 Trinder, *The Industrial Revolution in Shropshire,* p 117.

70 Hodge, J., *Richard Trevithick,* Botley, Oxford, Shire Publications, 1973, p 18.

engine capable of pulling a train of wagons along a railway.[71] This was so successful that before long 'locomotives' were hauling trains on a nation-wide network of railways, enabling the transport of goods and people to places far and wide. Within forty years there were two thousand miles of railway in Britain. The world had entered a new era of power, factories, transport and mobility.

Radical change was not confined to industry and, in the coming years, there were increasing demands for political reform and extension of the parliamentary franchise. The desire for reorganization was also being expressed in the medical profession. The practice of medical students arranging their own programme of lectures and hospital experience in London, as William had done, developed into structured courses covering the developing sciences, especially anatomy and chemistry. In 1815, the first legislation to distinguish trained practitioners from those who merely peddled quack remedies was passed by Parliament: this was the Apothecaries Act which required all new apothecary-surgeons to prove their competence by examination at the London Society of Apothecaries. Whereas Benjamin and William only had to persuade their masters that they were competent, their successors had to prove it by public examination. One Twentieth-Century writer on medical education called it an 'era of great individuals and low standards' and regretted that too many doctors were merely 'speculating in their studies' by learning the accumulated errors of the past, rather than 'reading the book of nature' by observation and experiment.[72] Medical students were dissolute, drunken and far from scholarly if Charles Dickens' character Bob Sawbones in the *Pickwick Papers* is typical. One contemporary writer said they were 'the most

---

71 Raistrick, A., *Dynasty of Ironfounders*, p 162.

72 Newman, C., *The Evolution of Medical Education in the Nineteenth Century*, Oxford University Press, 1957, p 56.

bearish I have ever beheld in a mass'.[73] Yet they were only following the example of their superiors, not least the obese and lascivious Prince Regent, and when these 'Sawbones' entered the burgeoning medical market as new members of the profession they could rightly claim that they had been appropriately educated, which the competing army of quacks and empirics could not. Competition from such uneducated people angered the regular profession for two reasons: one was the reasonable claim that they were untrustworthy and dangerous, the other that these competitors were stealing the justifiable profits of those who had invested time and money in learning the business properly. Demands were voiced that medical education be better organised so that qualified members of the profession could easily be distinguished from impostors, and that quackery be made illegal. The necessary reforms took more than fifty years to achieve, during which time a new generation of doctors, including Edward and his young brother Benjamin, experienced extensive changes to their education and legal status.

We know nothing of Edward's schooling. At one time his brother Richard went to school locally in Little Wenlock, and William was a boarder at Adams grammar school at Newport fifteen miles away, so Edward probably did something similar. He may also have been taught by his father when time permitted, or by a local cleric, possibly Samuel Walter who preached in the tradition of Rev John Fletcher, the fiery revivalist vicar of Madeley.[74] By the age of fourteen Edward had to think about his career and although he could easily follow his father into the medical business he was tempted at one time by another option. In 1805 the nation had rejoiced at the Royal Navy's triumph at Trafalgar. The legend of Nelson's fatal victory would have made him a hero to any teenage boy like Edward but there

---

73 Newman, C., *The Evolution of Medical Education*, p 42.

74 Trinder, B., *The Industrial Revolution in Shropshire*, p 161.

was also a family connection with the Navy. In 1789, the crew of *HMS Bounty,* then stationed in the Pacific Ocean, mutinied against what they alleged was the unnecessarily harsh discipline imposed by their commander, Lieutenant Bligh — though they may simply have wanted to return to the balmy life-style of Tahiti where they had enjoyed time ashore. Bligh and some loyal members of the crew were cast adrift in an open boat in the vast Pacific Ocean and, after a remarkable journey, reached the Dutch East Indies before returning to Britain to report the mutiny. Determined to bring the mutineers to justice, the Admiralty sent *HMS Pandora* to find them under the command of Captain Edward Edwards — the benevolent uncle who had financed William's medical education. On her return voyage *Pandora* was wrecked on the uncharted Great Barrier Reef. After another remarkable journey, the resourceful Captain Edwards returned to Britain with the surviving members of his crew and some of the mutineers only to be court-martialled for loss of his ship. This only slightly blunted his career, however, and he was subsequently promoted to the rank of Admiral of the White (now Vice-Admiral). The teenage Edward may have been tempted to emulate his heroic but ill-fated great-uncle but he decided to follow his father into the medical profession and became his apprentice at the age of fourteen. Edward's uncle Richard commented in a letter to William that 'It would have been a pity if he had gone to sea, and I was somewhat anxious in my wishes to prevent it'.[75] The context of this letter suggests that Edward had indeed considered extending his experience as a surgeon's mate in the navy.

Edward thus committed himself to the medical profession. He would already have been familiar with the shop in the family house and had probably taken an interest in his father's business from an early age; now he would have to acquire the knowledge and skills of an apothecary in earnest. As apprentice he would do the tidying,

---

75 Letter 4b, SA 1987/56/24., 30 June 1814.

cleaning, bottle washing and floor-sweeping before learning about the medicines, ointments and pills, weighing the ingredients and preparing them according to prescriptions and recipes written in Latin. Although he had studied the language at school, he now had to understand abbreviated instructions such as this:

> R. Aq. Ceraf. Nig. Cinnamon, āā oz iij. Syr & tinct. Croc. āā oz j. confect. alkerm *dr iij. spir. lavend. Comp. oz fs. sal. volat. oleof. dr ij S. julap.*[76]

The following, a favourite prescription for Gout of the famous Dr Sydenham, written in English, would have been a little easier though the measurements were rather less precise:

> *Take of the Roots of Horseradish sliced three ounces; of Garden Scurvy-grass twelve Handfuls; of water-Cresses, and Brooklime, of Sage and Mint, each four handfuls; The Peels of six Oranges, two Nutmegs bruised; of* Brunswick Mum[77] *twelve pints: Distil them in a common Still and draw only six pints of Water for use.*[78]

Edward would also have to deal with patients in the shop, hear their stories and assess their symptoms, though this would rarely require

---

76 In Shaw, P., *A New Practice of Physic,* London Longman, 1738. This seemingly impenetrable instruction indicates the nature and form of ingredients required, eg *cinnamon water*, the quantities, eg *oz iii* (3 ounces), *dr iii* (3 drachms), *oz fs* (half an ounce), or *aa* (in equal parts). Amazingly, this kind of formula was still being used as late as the 1960s.

77 A kind of beer brewed from wheat malt and flavoured with aromatic herbs, originally made at Brunswick in Germany. OED On-line edition accessed 26/3/2013. Distillation would reduce the volume to 6 pints.

78 *The Whole Works of that Excellent Practical Physician, Dr Thomas Sydenham, tenth edition corrected from the original Latin by John Pechey MD.* London, 1734.

more than an inspection of a wound or rash, feeling the pulse and observing the colour or pallor of the skin. His father would be there to teach him and, when the shop could be left unattended, they would go out together to visit patients.

After about two years' experience as an apprentice Edward embarked on six months' study in London. It must have been an exciting adventure for the sixteen-year old to exchange familiar Coalbrookdale for the boisterous, crowded capital. The family letters that survive from this period reveal something of Edward's character, the sacrifices his family made for his education and the delights and dangers of city life, which his relatives were at pains to warn him about. Edward began his London studies in the autumn of 1813 because the surgeons' private schools, although independent, conformed to the academic year of the universities. By this time his uncle Richard Edwards was living at 9 Great Russell Street in Bloomsbury, close to the British Museum, and it is likely that Edward lodged with him and certainly had his support. Richard wrote to his brother William:

> 'No doubt you will be greatly gratified to find Edward of so steady and careful a turn. Mrs Cave used to speak highly of him, and of his assiduity at lectures and Anatomy I think you can hardly have any idea. He is as regular as clockwork, and only wants to be not discomposed from his methodical manner.[79]

In London Edward would have to choose which courses to attend, being influenced by their reputation and what he could afford. The best teachers, who included the leading and most aspiring surgeons of the day, could earn hundreds of pounds from course fees despite intense competition to attract students. In Edward's time there were 250-300

---

79 SA, 1987/56/24, Letter, Richard to William, Jun 30 1814.

students attending the surgeons' courses and about fifty others studying with physicians, so there was also competition among students to get on the best courses.[80] The surgeons usually gave their lectures in their own houses where they also provided facilities for dissection. Finding enough subjects to dissect was a problem and recourse sometimes had to be made to the 'body-snatchers' and 'resurrection men' who would find the necessary materials from recent burials in return for a generous financial consideration and no questions asked. Students could attend as many courses as they could afford or find time for, as well as the many free lectures given by surgeons for the benefit of an increasingly curious public as a way of advertising their professional existence. These public lectures were often held in one of the city coffee-houses where commercial and financial transactions also took place and where physicians made themselves available for consultation by apothecaries on behalf of their patients.

Because the courses were organised individually rather than as a co-ordinated curriculum, the students had to construct their own timetables. They would also have to find time for clinical experience by 'walking the wards', and for travel between the various places they attended — on foot because there were no omnibuses and they were unlikely to spend money on sedan chairs. Walking the wards involved observing a surgeon as he attended his patients in the hospital or dispensary, watching operations and, if possible, spending time as a 'dresser' carrying out treatments according to the surgeons' instructions. Students could therefore study all day if they wished. A typical timetable for an enthusiastic student is shown in Table 4.1.[81]

---

80 Lawrence, S., *Charitable Knowledge: hospital pupils and practitioners in eighteenth century London,* Cambridge University Press, 1996, p 111.

81 Lawrence, S. *Charitable Knowledge*, p 172.

Table 4.1

A typical student's lecture timetable

7.30 — 9.0 am	*Materia medica* or medicine
9.00 — 10.0	Chemistry
10.30 — 11.30	Midwifery
11.30 — 1.00	Clinical observations at Hospital or Dispensary
2.00 — 3.00 pm	Anatomy
3.00-5.00	Dissection
5.00-6.00	Midwifery and women's diseases
7.00-8.00 or 8.00-9.00	Surgery

Plus reading text-books and notes taken at lectures

The hospitals attended by the students were those at which many physicians and surgeons held honorary appointments. These 'Voluntary Subscription Hospitals' were so called because they were funded by large numbers of people who 'voluntarily subscribed' small annual sums, rather than by one or more grand donors or by the taxpayer. They originated in the Eighteenth and early Nineteenth centuries to care for the 'deserving poor', meaning those people who could not afford to pay for their treatment but were not so destitute as to qualify for parish support under the Poor Laws which was seen as shameful. In Edward's time, there were seven such hospitals in London: Guy's, The London, St George's, The Westminster, The Middlesex and the much older St Thomas's and St Bartholomew's which had adopted the new Voluntary Subscription system. All of them eventually established their own medical schools. The patients accepted that they would be used as teaching material for students as *quid pro quo* for being admitted free of charge. As well as walking the wards at these hospitals, students could get experience at numerous out-patient dispensaries that were funded by a similar charitable system. These were simple affairs without facilities for further investigations, because, in the days before careful examination, laboratory tests and X-rays, doctors only broadly identified the disease and prescribed medicines that were hardly more than palliative. But they were places where newcomers to the profession could gain experience and, just as importantly, where doctors could meet and discuss ideas about disease, assess their treatments and learn from their activities — and their mistakes. Students flocked to London to study and Edward was fortunate to do so at a time when his profession was entering a period of profound change. In the provinces, where most doctors lived and worked, there were few opportunities for them to meet but, in the hospitals, dispensaries and lecture rooms of London, all sorts of ideas, rumours and frustrations could be aired.

Moves to reform the profession did not originate only in hospitals and lecture rooms. Discontent had been voiced for many years and came to a head, albeit temporarily, in the 1790s. Whereas the apothecaries' traditional role was only to dispense the prescriptions of physicians, by the end of the Eighteenth Century they had become the doctors for people unable to afford the high fees of physicians, but still earned their money by selling medicines not by charging for attendance. Yet they had no monopoly in this market and a new kind of shopkeeper had arisen, the 'chemists and druggists' who sold proprietary medicines but made no pretensions to proper diagnosis. The regular apothecaries, who believed that an Act of 1748 had given them the monopoly of supplying medicines, sought to suppress competition from such alleged interlopers who were said to be imperfectly trained in the necessary skills and therefore a danger to the public.[82] In 1794, two hundred apothecaries assembled at London's Crown and Anchor Tavern to protest, claiming that they were losing as much as £200 a year to the

---

82 Bell, Jacob and Redwood, Theophilus, *Historical Sketch of the Progress of Pharmacy*, London, The Pharmaceutical Society of Great Britain, 1880, p 33.

druggists. They founded the General Pharmaceutical Association of Great Britain to demand legal protection from unqualified competitors. At this time the Royal College of Physicians and the Society of Apothecaries had power to inspect apothecaries' premises in London but there had never been any attempt to regulate medical practitioners elsewhere. The new General Pharmaceutical Association wanted to extend such regulation nationwide and proposed two ways to do so: firstly, to persuade the druggists to trade only in the wholesale market and not directly with the public; secondly, to 'restrain ignorant and unqualified persons from practising at all', which would require a means of distinguishing trained persons from the untrained.[83] This was the first call for reform of the profession, a process that would eventually last sixty years, but despite its grand-sounding title and earnest objectives the Association achieved little and soon vanished from the scene.

With so many people offering medical services — physicians, surgeons, apothecaries, druggists, proprietary medicine makers, empirics and quacks — there was a lively market in cures, in which it was impossible to distinguish the honest from the sham or the genuine from the fraud. Following the brief existence of the General Pharmaceutical Association, demands for a nationwide system to exclude 'ignorant persons' from medical practice gradually increased. A flurry of excitement amongst apothecaries erupted following the 1802 Medicines Act, which increased the 'Stamp Duty' on proprietary medicines, a tax that had been introduced in 1783 along with taxes on many other commodities such as tobacco, spirits, glass, bricks and tea. The tax was a revenue-raising exercise of which apothecaries approved because it raised the prices of their competitors. But the Medicines Act was so imprecisely worded that, although apothecaries were exempt from it, it appeared to apply to their 'own-brand' medicines not sold or advertised elsewhere. Thus if a shopkeeper sold a widely available

---

83 Bell, J., and Redwood, T., *Historical Sketch of the Progress of Pharmacy*, p 34-7.

brand of lozenges the label would carry the 'Government Stamp' to show that tax had been paid. No tax was due if, after consultation, an apothecary prescribed his own-make lozenges but, if a customer specifically asked for the same lozenges without consultation, the sale would appear to be taxable. People who suspected tax was thus being evaded were encouraged to tell the authorities, thereby exposing apothecaries to prosecution. The 1802 Act was amended in 1803 to clarify the position, but the confusion had raised the question of how to distinguish a legitimate provider of medical care from druggists and others medicine-sellers, such as bookshops and newspaper proprietors. As yet there was no legal definition of a medical practitioner and, although apothecaries had to complete a formal apprenticeship, anyone could sell medicines and even call himself a surgeon without having had any training.

The Royal College of Physicians was concerned because of its legal duty to supervise apothecaries' shops, so, in 1804, Dr John Latham, a prominent fellow of the College and later its president, proposed a new and more radical scheme of regulation. The country would be divided into sixteen districts in each of which a physician would be appointed to investigate the credentials of every physician, surgeon, apothecary, chemist, druggist and medicine seller in his district. The findings in each county would be reported to the relevant Quarter Sessions or Summer Assize which were then the local-government authorities.[84] This grandiose, dogmatic and probably unworkable scheme was never implemented but it did encourage the College of Physicians to consider how medical practice might be better regulated. A more sensible plan was proposed by Dr Edward Harrison and his colleagues in Lincolnshire, based on proper evidence of the extent to which untrained practitioners were operating. His report to the College of Physicians in 1806, which had the support of many eminent people in London, proposed a way for Parliament to bring order and higher

---

84 Loudon, I., *Medical Care and the General Practitioner, 1750-1850,* p 139.

standards to the profession and make untrained practice illegal. Central to his proposals was education. For each section of the profession there would be minimum periods of training and a minimum age at which newly qualified practitioners would be allowed to start work. Non-compliance would render offenders liable to prosecution. The College rejected Harrison's proposals but they had taken the apothecaries' demands a stage further and stimulated a debate about how the different sections of the profession should be educated and licensed.

Though Harrison's attempt to involve the College of Physicians failed, the apothecaries were spurred into further action for a different reason — another huge increase in a tax. In its efforts to pay for years of war in America and Europe the government had imposed taxes on anything that could be measured, including, in 1798, a tax on personal incomes over £60 (said to be only temporary!). The tax burden was heavy for everyone but, after the rate of the glass-tax was raised five-fold, apothecaries felt especially aggrieved because of their extensive use of glass bottles. In 1812, 160 apothecaries rallied to protest at this imposition, again at the Crown and Anchor Tavern. Such was their mood that other lingering grievances were raised and a new group was formed to defend their interests.[85] At first this new Association of Apothecaries and Surgeon Apothecaries was available only to Londoners because travel from the provinces was expensive and impracticable but, as its importance was realised, membership was soon extended to the rest of England and Wales. A plan was to be put to Parliament 'for improving and protecting the profession of Apothecary, Surgeon-Apothecary and Practitioner of Midwifery in England and Wales' and support was sought from the London Society of Apothecaries and the Royal Colleges.[86] The government was prepared to accept the plan but the colleges were not and the

---

85 Newman, C., *The Evolution of Medical Education,* p 65.

86 Newman, C., *The Evolution of Medical Education,* p 67.

legislation eventually placed the burden of regulation solely, and therefore reluctantly, on the Society of Apothecaries. One effect of this was to make the titles 'Apothecary', and 'Surgeon Apothecary' out of date. These doctors were popular among their customer-patients because they could do almost everything: the three skills of 'physic' comprising medicine, surgery *and* pharmacy. The cumbersome titles were abandoned in favour of the simpler but non-specific 'general' practitioner — but that is for later in this story.

All this was going on while Edward was studying in London and he and his fellow students probably debated the various ideas that would shape their future and the way they would earn their livings. He had applied himself assiduously to his studies and, despite being warned not to fall into worldly temptations, he must have seen something of metropolitan life. But he was needed at home. By March 1814 he had been in London for six months and would soon obtain his certificates of attendance. William meanwhile was working very hard, though he rather hoped to get a little help from his younger son Richard, now thirteen years old, who, he said, 'could do a great Deal in the Shop if he was willing, but is generally very idle and fond of play'.[87] This was perhaps not surprising since his home-work was reading the First Book of Caesar. William regretted he couldn't let Edward stay in London longer but his resources were limited because they depended on the dwindling prosperity of his patients who worked in the struggling iron industry. A second course of Chemistry would have cost another £20 'which is a considerable sum in the present state of my affairs' but Edward would be able to 'make up the deficiency by reading'. However, William held out the possibility of a return to London at a later date 'if Stocks continue to advance as rapidly as they have'. He said that Mr Brookes (one of the most popular and respected teachers between 1800 and 1820) undertook to teach his pupils Anatomy in three months

---

87 SA, 1987/56/15, Letter, William to Edward, 22 Feb 1814.

for a fee of £50, board included,[88] which was a much better deal than he had had as a student himself. He told Edward that if he returned to London in future:

> I think you will have many more advantages than I had as I had no one to consult in any difficult case without making it extremely unpleasant. You will have time to see Operations at the different hospitals which you will no doubt turn to much advantage, and I hope you will not think me unnecessarily penurious when you consider how I am situated.[89]

The winter was severe and fuel costly:

> We have generally had a fire in the Back Kitchen during the severe weather for the servants and the children to sit and be washed by, which I prefer to [having one in] the Shop or Parlour.

The chimney in the shop smoked badly and gave extra work to the servants and William and Elizabeth could manage without a fire in the Parlour — no central heating fuelled by North Sea Gas in William's time. The weather was so cold in London that a Frost Fair was held on the frozen Thames (it was the last one because milder winters, the demolition of the many-arched London Bridge and the construction of the Embankment subsequently prevented the river from freezing). In 1814 the ice was so thick that an elephant was led onto it without breaking it and crowds of people thronged the many stalls and entertainment booths in the Fair. The very idea that Edward

---

88 SA, 1987/56/15, Letter, William to Edward, 22 Feb 1814.

89 SA, 1987/56/15, Letter, William to Edward, 22 Feb 1814.

might have followed the elephant onto the perilous ice worried his mother:

> Your mother has been afraid of the ice breaking with you on the Thames.

Elizabeth seems to have been very anxious for her son, far away in a city she had probably never visited herself. William added:

> 'Yr Mother was afraid you was [sic] one of the two who were lost during the late conflagration at the Custom House, till you convinced her to the contrary'.

Why Edward rather than any of the other 1.2 million people in London should have been present at the Custom House is unclear but mothers rightly worry about their children.

It was not only fires and frost fairs that Edward was enjoined to avoid. The family's religious attitudes were somewhat puritanical:

> You should do very well not to spend your time and Money at Plays etc, they are foolish empty Nonsense and only for idle dissipated Characters, beneath the Notice of any man of Sense and Business and frequently lead young people into bad Connections.

The next sentence in this affectionate and newsy letter at Christmas time ends it rather abruptly:

> Mr Cureton is drinking Tea here, Mrs Locock is ill of Rheumatism.
> Wishing you the Compts of the Season, not too late
> Remains etc, Wm Edwards

The letters to Edward are full of family and local news much of which seems unimportant now. William tells Edward about his grandmother Frances Wright: 'Your grandmother is expected daily at Mrs Yate's [Edward's cousin] during her approaching Accouchment [*sic*]' and writes about his uncle Peter Wright (P.W.), Aunt Fanny Yate and cousin Ann Bancks: 'Mr P.W. is embonpoint,[90] it is a trade not likely to fail you. Mrs Hall, late Miss A. Bancks idem [*the same*]'. Obesity is not a problem new in the Twenty-First Century, it seems.

William took advantage of Edward being in London to discuss medical instruments and books and to advise him on his purchases. Edward had bought a catheter and some obstetric forceps but rather regretted it (or his father had disapproved of such extravagance as he already had a good set):

> I think the best thing to do with [them] is to prevail upon the Maker to exchange them for a pocket case [of instruments], almost on any terms and it will be better to buy a set of Tooth Instruments ... and Midwifery Instmnts [*sic*] are very seldom necessary.

Edward was told about what books to buy for his father and for the practice:

> I could wish you to buy Celsus's works in Latin, if you can meet with them cheap, they are the best works on Medical Subjects in Latin, and would improve you in the Language; or Hippocrates with Galen's comments.

In another letter Edward is advised:

---

90 Embonpoint: Plumpness, well-nourished appearance of body: in complimentary or euphemistic sense. OED, online edition.

> If you begin with the old Authors you will not want any new ones for some time: I should like the Celsus at seven or 9 shillings & the little work by Dr Clarke if you think it worth your Money, which, however, I can assure you is very scarce, too much to be laid out in Books, unless such are absolutely necessary.[91]

Textbooks in Latin were all very well but William's liking for the 'old authors' was at odds with the rapid changes in medical science occurring at this time, of which William was apparently unaware. Keeping up to date in medicine was difficult even then.

Edward may have had other ideas than returning to Coalbrookdale despite his father's financial difficulties and need for help. Many young men who had gone to London for their education were excited and challenged by the intellectual and professional climate, even if they eschewed theatre-going and 'bad connections', and Edward was similarly tempted to remain there. Many others such as William Marsden and Langdon Down, both near contemporaries of Edward's, stayed in London and became eminent in their fields. Edward may also have worried about how he would fit into the family on his return. He was moving from adolescence into adulthood and would have to live in the same house as his parents and five siblings. Family tensions would not have been surprising in such a crowded household.

He overcame these doubts, however, when William reassured him of his future independence:

> As you appear desirous of taking an active part in the Business on your return, it will be right that you have every necessary Accommodation to enable you to attain so laudable a Pursuit with satisfaction to you and your

---

91 SA, 1987/56/16, Letter, William to Edward, 7 Mar 1814.

Friends, & if I may judge from what has occurred during your Absence, you will have sufficient Employment without concerning yourself with domestic Affairs.[92]

A little later William wrote:

You seem to have given up all thought of a Situation in Town, you must therefore endeavour to be as comfortable as possible as you can at home which can only be done by each party bearing and forbearing.

One of Edward's concerns had been how the garden would be managed. There was only a small garden around their house but on the other side of the road they had developed some land bordered by the Upper Furnace Pool. William said he would be happy for Edward to do what he liked there because if he, William, was to pay for it someone in the family would need to superintend it as 'the generality of servants is not to be trusted'. Edward would have time to do so because he would be less busy than his father, and William said it would be a pity to give it up after 'laying out so much money in the Improvements'. More importantly, there was a concern about the proposed division of labour, both professionally and domestically: Edward was to manage the shop, leaving his father free to visit the patients in their homes, but the shop was in the house which was his mother's domain. So who would be in charge, and who would do what? William replied:

Your mother thinks it unkind that you should express so much anxiety about her interfering in the Shop. That will be your Province & the House is hers, there is no necessity for one Department encroaching on another, but as the Shop is a thoroughfare to the House people

---

92 SA, 1987/56/15, Letter, William to Edward, 22 Feb 1814.

must unavoidably come through the Shop Door with Bread & Meat, but I do not see that that can materially interrupt you either in your Studies or Business especially where persons are peaceably disposed & without which no family can be comfortable.[93]

William closed the letter by saying:

'Your Mother has a Cold, Earache &c. the rest are tolerably well ...

I remain Dr Edward,
Your affectionate Father
Wm Edwards
P.S. Your mother desires me to add that you will be at Liberty to clean the Shop in your own way if you prefer it to the present method; & to have a fire when you think it necessary.

'Keep clean your shops in eminent degree', as the apothecary poet had said.

Edward returned to Coalbrookdale. Since he was due to receive his certificates of attendance on 25th March 1814, his father told him not to prolong his stay in London 'as it cannot be done without additional Expense'. He expected to see Edward 'about the 27th March' because if he stayed longer 'the busy season' would be over. William gave ample advice about the journey. He said the coaches from Shropshire usually called at the 'Green Man and Still' tavern in Oxford Street, and Edward should take a coach from there to Worcester and thence to Ironbridge, and walk the remaining mile. That would be better than travelling on the Shrewsbury coach which stopped at Shifnal five miles away where it

---

93 SA 1987/56/16, Letter, William to Edward, 7 Mar 1814.

would be more difficult to collect his luggage. Expense was important: 'I would not have you come by the Mail as that is more expensive, & they are very shy of luggage'. Payment for excess baggage cost money even then. There remained the matter of clothing, for travelling outside on the coach to minimise the fare would expose him to the cold of an inclement March. But money was short, and Edward's time in London had been expensive:

> We have suffered many privations on your account, particularly in the Articles of Clothing, the Winter being so severe, and I am afraid you have felt the want of a Great Coat, indeed mine is very shabby and it is too cold to ride long journeys without.

William said that by travelling outside on the coach Edward would save enough money to buy a coat which would certainly be necessary for the following winter when he would be visiting patients. A 'bottle green Beaver will not cost much', said William, but 'be sure to have it made large enough'.

So Edward returned to join the business and manage the shop in familiar Coalbrookdale. He left London at a crucial time: an end to the prolonged war in Europe and overseas was agreed by the Treaty of Fontainbleau but pressure was mounting for social and political reform in Britain. And for Edward there were changes in both his family and his profession which would reach far into his future.

Chapter 5

William and Edward

Edward's return to Coalbrookdale was welcomed by everyone. His mother was freed from the fear that Edward would fall into the freezing Thames or die in a house fire, while his father had his help in the shop and was spared the cost of his studies in London. His sister Betsey, now sixteen, would surely be glad to have her brother's companionship, and his brothers Richard and William, now twelve and nine respectively, could resume their boyish games with him. His younger sisters Fanny and Anna Maria, aged four, would want to hear all about their big brother's London adventures.

By now Rose Hill was fully occupied by William and Elizabeth, their two grown-up children Betsey and Edward, the two young boys and the younger girls. In 1815, a baby daughter Mary was born but joy turned to sorrow when she died soon afterwards. Such grief is not easily resolved, but in 1816 the family rejoiced again in the birth of another child, named Benjamin after his grandfather, who was destined to be the fourth Coalbrookdale doctor. A family of this kind would have had servants, probably a cook and a maid with a stable lad or groom to look after the horse and grounds. The children would go to one of the schools in the Dale run by the philanthropic Darby family and, later, the boys at least, to grammar schools at Shifnal or Newport. By now Edward was firmly committed to being a doctor but such a career was not available to Betsey because she was a woman and, let's imagine, a pretty one. This was the period so vividly described by Jane Austen in *Pride and Prejudice*. If her well-known assertion that 'a single man possessed of good fortune must be in want of a wife'[94], how much more would an impecunious single woman be in need of a husband? Like the daughters in Austen's

---

94 The 'universally acknowledged truth' in the opening sentence of *Pride and Prejudice*

Bennett family, the Edwards were respectable but would not expect to inherit even a modest fortune and there were no rich bachelors or dashing soldiers in Coalbrookdale. It was an industrial village populated by miners, smiths and tradesmen, and only a few families could have provided an appropriate suitor. There may have been some eligible young men in the area but, whether by choice or lack of a proposal, Betsey never found her single man of good fortune. Nor did her brother Edward find a bride and they both remained single, living at Rose Hill with their mother, brothers and sisters. Their home was a busy one, full of people fulfilling their various roles: seeing patients in the shop or visiting them on foot or horseback, housekeeping, supervising the servants, going to school, doing Latin homework, having music lessons and playing childish games. And after his work Edward could once again enjoy the spacious garden by the Pool in contrast to the noisy bustle of London.

Family life for the Edwards was comfortable by the standards of the time, despite their financial constraints. They were on familiar terms with the educated members of the community, including the proprietors and managers of the Coalbrookdale Company, especially the Darbys with whom they occasionally 'took tea'. They also had relatives in the Dale, their cousins the Morgans and the Yates, grandchildren of Benjamin Wright, and they would meet their neighbours at church or the Quaker Meeting House. Twenty-First Century people would certainly find the conditions of the Edwards's family home inconvenient with its cold and draughty rooms lit at night by candles and lacking a bath and water-closet but, by comparison with labouring folk, they were comfortable. In some ways, however, the less genteel inhabitants of the Dale were also well situated because the Coalbrookdale Company organised a variety of skilled occupations for the growing population, such as the mill (managed by the Morgan family), the school, the shops and a laundry. But with only scanty transport this was still a relatively isolated community, unlike nearby Shrewsbury or Wellington which developed around ancient markets and had various established industries. With the completion of the Iron Bridge a new settlement arose around it that attracted many businesses from Madeley and it soon became a town in its own right, eponymously called Ironbridge, and though the bridge made it easier to get to the markets and shops in Broseley, that town was already in decline.

The social values and behaviour of the community were greatly influenced by attitudes to religion. From time to time there were 'revivals' of religious fervour, though backsliding was common where the lot of many was low-paid physical labour. In the last years of the Eighteenth Century and especially in wartime, Methodism had a large following and, in the 1780s, had been closely associated with the parish church in Madeley where the evangelical priest John Fletcher was vicar. The enthusiastic preacher Samuel Taylor led revival campaigns in and around Coalbrookdale, converting 'precious souls from sin to holiness', and successive revivals occurred in 1803, 1814 and 1822.[95] The Anglican church in Madeley, however, was not well attended. In 1799 there were fewer than thirty communicants, the incumbent did not even live in the parish[96] and, when a new church was opened not far away in Malinslee, the church in Madeley became neglected. The Edwards family was nominally Anglican (William often wrote of his regret at being unable to go to church because of his demanding work) although they were sympathetic to the previous religious observations of Benjamin Wright and his Quaker Friends. William's brother Richard, an Anglican clergyman himself, wrote to him in 1818 suggesting he might display his Quaker allegiance more openly by means of his headwear:

> I have wondered why you never wear a broad-brimmed hat as old Mr Wright did, living as you do among Quakers. Edward told me he would attend the Quaker meeting

---

95 Trinder, B., *The Industrial Revolution in Shropshire,* p 198.

96 Trinder, B., *The Industrial Revolution in Shropshire,* p 174.

[in London], which would be as profitable to him as to attend the London Hospitals.[97]

This brotherly comment may have been made at least partly in jest but it does suggest that William had an affinity for the Quakers and was not merely 'living among' them, and it certainly indicates a degree of religious commitment.

For all the relative comfort and convenience of their lives, the Edwards family ultimately depended for their livelihood on the economy of the Dale which, in turn, was based on hazardous work in mines and foundries. For the miners, whether of coal or iron, wages for a physically demanding life in which danger and tragedy were always present were low, especially in the Shropshire mines — £1/1s for a 72 hour week, or less than 2d an hour.[98] The 'Rules for the Preservation of Good Order' of William Reynolds and Co. (as the old Coalbrookdale Company was then called) in the early 1800s stated that all workers must be in their 'proper places from six in the morning until six in the evening (breakfast and dinner excepted)'.[99] In winter-time, therefore, the miners would not see the light of day for a whole week as they walked to and from the mines. To enter the pit they were lowered for hundreds of feet down the shaft in baskets, or clinging dangerously to loops in a long rope. At the coalface they had to work by the feeble light of naked candle-flames, at least until 1815 when Sir Humphry Davy invented the safety lamp, though even this vital improvement was ignored for years in many mines. The miners crouched in tunnels less than three feet high, hacking away the coal and rock a few inches at a time.[100] It is hard enough work to swing a pick-axe standing up,

---

97 SA 1987/56/1, Letter, Richard Edwards (senior) William Edwards (senior).

98 Trinder, B., *The Industrial Revolution in Shropshire*, p 203.

99 Raistrick, A., *A Dynasty of Ironfounders: the Darbys of Coalbrookdale*, Appendix 8

100 Trinder, B., *The Industrial Revolution in Shropshire,* p 210.

but to crouch in a low tunnel and swing it from side to side must have been very arduous indeed. After the coal and unwanted rubble had been loosened, it had to be removed which was the work of boys as young as ten or even younger. Coal and waste were loaded onto sledges and dragged by children crawling on all fours to a wider part of the tunnel, whence it was transferred to the main shaft in pony-carts and from there hoisted to the surface.[101] In 1772 John Fletcher, who as vicar of Madeley must have known the miners well, described their working conditions:

> In these low and dreary vaults, all the elements seemed combined against them. Destructive damps, and clouds of noxious dust, infect the air they breathe. Sometimes water incessantly distils on their naked bodies; or bursting upon them in streams, drowns them or deluges their work. At other times, pieces of detached rocks crush them to death; or the earth, breaking in upon them, buries them alive. And frequently sulphureous vapours, kindled in an instant by the light of their candles, form subterraneous thunder and lightning.[102]

These were the conditions in which men and boys, children even, toiled in the pits for long hours every day except Sundays. They must have been thankful to survive each day, not knowing what might befall them the next day on return to those 'dreary vaults'. An event in 1810 at the Madeley Meadow Pit illustrates the danger to everyone who worked underground. Thirteen men and eight ponies were working at a depth of 210 yards when fire broke out, possibly ignited by a candle, but by great good fortune all the men and ponies were rescued. The next

---

[101] Trinder, B., *The Industrial Revolution in Shropshire*, p 210.

[102] Rev, John Fletcher, *An Appeal to a Matter of Fact and Common Sense*, quoted in Trinder, B., *The Industrial Revolution in Shropshire*, p 210.

day four men went down to examine the damage but, according to the accident report, 'there was too much sulphur and all were suffocated'. It was said that:

> The situation of the poor widows and fatherless children may be more easily conceived than described. One widow was pregnant, 19 children from four families were 'left to implore their fathers' sudden and unexpected deaths'.[103]

Such tragedies were common, and must have produced plenty of work for the Coalbrookdale doctors. Most accidents were due to collapse of the tunnels but nearly half the deaths were caused by falling down the vertical mine-shafts. Between 1801 and 1819 there were 355 deaths in East Shropshire mines, and, in the next ten years, another 236 men were killed — an average of twenty a year, or one every two or three weeks.[104] Accidents could also occur on the surface, when boilers burst or gunpowder stores exploded. In September 1801, a torrential rainstorm flooded the Upper Furnace Pool and breached the dam. The Old Furnace lay only a few yards below the dam and when the flood burst upon the molten ore and burning coke there was a huge explosion and widespread wreckage. One witness said '... the furnace and blowing mill, the pool and dam and the buildings are all gone'.[105] Incredibly, though the water rushed on further down the hill causing more damage, there were no deaths or injuries. Accidents and loss of life of this kind, whether above or below ground, were good reasons for the Darby family, steeped in their Quaker philanthropy, to provide cottages for the widows of their workers because there was no Social

---

103 Ironbridge Gorge Museum Trust, Information Sheet No 6.

104 Trinder, B., *The Industrial Revolution in Shropshire,* p 211.

105 Raistrick, A., *Dynasty of Ironfounders: the Darbys of Coalbrookdale,* p 227.

Security. It would have been part of William and Edwards duties to come to the aid of those unfortunate people too. No medicine would have prevented the deaths or cured the injuries, but the suffering of the wounded and bereaved would have exercised their skill and compassion within the limited methods then available.

Such were the circumstances of life in Coalbrookdale in the early years of the Nineteenth Century. Further afield, by 1814, the war seemed to be at an end and it was hoped that the peace negotiated at the Treaty of Fontainbleau would allow the iron industry to recover. Napoleon's escape from Elba renewed the conflict until his eventual defeat at Waterloo in 1815, which at last ensured peace after forty years of intermittent war. But the sense of relief that comes with victory did not lift the economic depression and social distress. As production was transferred to more efficient factories many people were thrown out of their accustomed work and even the lucky ones, who kept their jobs, found their wages reduced. In Coalbrookdale where wages were lower than in other iron-working areas:[106] '… haggard hunger, despairing wretchedness … and armed ruffians' were abroad again. The Edwards family must have seen the distress of the people around them and shared their misfortunes, to some extent at least. Many years before the National Health Service where medical care is free at the point of use, if the price of 'Physic', or medicine, rose beyond what people could afford, there would be no money to provide the incomes of the doctors who prescribed it.

While economic difficulties engulfed the iron trade and its dependent services there was another challenge to the medical businesses of men like William and Edward. By the early Nineteenth Century a flourishing market had been established in propriety medicines that innumerable advertisements claimed could both prevent and cure disease. Hundreds of products were available whose makers described their prodigious efficacy in advertisements that borrowed heavily from the terminology

---

[106] Trinder, B., *The Industrial Revolution in Shropshire*, p 203.

of orthodox practitioners. The proprietors often claimed a spurious authenticity by prefixing their names with the title of 'doctor'. For example, 'Dr' Solomon's Celebrated Medicines promised to cure 'scorbutic eruptions, scrophulous or venereal taint and ... consumptive habits'; and 'Dr' Sibley's Re-animating Solar Tincture' was claimed to be 'the best medicine for Debility, Consumption, Nervous and Rheumatic complaints, spasms ...' and much more. Dicey and Co. of London sold several brands such Bateman's Pectoral Drops (good for coughs, agues, fevers and even rheumatism), Anderson's True Scots Pills (promotes digestion and relieves bilious headaches) and Betton's British Oil whose 'superior efficiency is too well known to require any comment, Price 1s 9d'. Godfrey's Cordial was very good for getting children to sleep but contained so much opium that sometimes the children never woke again.

To the undiscerning purchaser these medicines would appear to be every bit as good as the doctors' prescriptions and much easier to obtain because there was no need to visit the apothecary or pay for his 'journey'. The advertisements implied that the medicines they advertised were better than the doctors' ineffective potions and they offered supporting evidence: sorry tales of men and women who had been ineffectively treated by the regular doctors — until, by good fortune, they heard of the relevant remedy and were rapidly cured. For example, in one such testimonial, Richard Partridge said he had 'placed himself under the care of a medical gentleman whose efforts proved ineffectual' but was cured as soon as he started taking Owen's British Drops. Another man, known only as J. R., who had been suffering for a year from 'a certain disorder' said that:

> After being under the treatment of several professional gentlemen for a great length of time they reduced me nearly to death's door by the use of mercurials &c...

> Finding their endeavours all in vain I despaired of ever being cured.

He was then advised by 'a friend' to take Owens British Drops which contained Barbados Tar and turpentine, and 'was really lost with astonishment at the wonderful improvements'. After taking three more bottles of this remarkable medicine he was 'soundly cured'.

The makers of these products claimed that their medicines were safer than those of the doctors because they did not contain poisonous metals such as mercury, antimony and lead that the doctors prescribed.[107] Like the proprietary medicine makers, the new 'general practitioners' who were emerging from the chrysalis of the old apothecaries still had to make their money from selling medicines because, by law, they were not allowed to charge for 'giving advice', that is, for diagnosing disease and prescribing treatment. This was because over a hundred years earlier, in 1705, the Royal College of Physicians had sued an apothecary called Rose, alleging that he was acting illegally by 'giving advice', which was the duty of physicians.[108] The case went as far as the House of Lords where, in favour of the physicians, it was established that, although apothecaries were commonly consulted on medical matters and often did give advice, they were not legally entitled to charge for doing so. Their Lordships also decided, in favour of the apothecaries that, because the situation could not be reversed and people could buy any medicine from any source they chose, apothecaries should be allowed

---

107 This was not always true, according to *The Lancet*. Spilsbuy's Antiscorbutic drops consisted of mercuric chloride antimony and alcohol as well as orange and gentian; Ford's Balsam of Horehound contained opium in brandy, with liquorice, horehound and plenty of honey; and Plimmer's Pills had both mercurous chloride and antimony. Dalby's carminative had opium, spirits of wine and caraway, asafoetida and peppermint; and that great stand-by, Daffy's Elixir, had opium and proof spirit with flavouring of santile wood shaving, elecampane root, aniseed, caraway coriander, liquorice and raisins. *The Lancet, 1823, p 62.*

108 Loudon, I., *Medical Care and the General Practitioner, 1750-1850*, p 22

to give advice so long as they did not charge for it. Therefore they had no choice but to make their money from preparing and selling medicines. So, for example, when Benjamin Wright visited John Onions he could not charge for the knowledge or skill on which he based his diagnosis but could charge 1s 6d for the time taken to go to his home, as well as 2s 0d for a mixture and 1s 0d for a tincture which he prescribed. Apothecaries were therefore upstaged by the thriving proprietary-medicine trade because the makers did not undergo long and expensive training, could mass-produce their medicines cheaply and did not spend time with their customers in making decisions. In the coming years, dissatisfaction with this inadequate medico-legal compromise ran parallel to demands for reform in politics and industry though it was not so violently expressed as in those fields. Because there was no professional association for the majority of practitioners, there was no outlet for their frustration and no means of debating possible remedies for a state of affairs that they claimed was not only a threat to their honest livelihood but a danger to the public too.

The few medical journals that then existed did not usually carry correspondence or discussion about concerns of this kind, and national newspapers were expensive and not readily available in Shropshire (while Edward was in London, William sometimes asked him to send second-hand copies 'if the price was right'). The penny post had not yet made letters affordable and travel was slow, expensive and impracticable, so it was almost impossible to develop a consensus of interested parties. A powerful stimulus was therefore needed, which eventually arose from the threat to personal incomes as a result of an increase in the tax on glass, which, of course, apothecaries used for medicine bottles. In 1812 a great meeting of apothecaries was held at the Crown and Anchor Tavern in London, ostensibly to protest at this unreasonable imposition, and this meeting gave them the opportunity to express their other grievances. It was agreed that the out-dated tripartite system of physician, surgeon and apothecary should be abolished in favour of a united profession, or at least of a degree of co-operation between the medical Royal Colleges and Society of Apothecaries in the regulation of medical practice. Until then the authority of those bodies was only valid within seven miles of London, but for the great majority of the profession who worked in the provinces there had never been any form of regulation at all. The new general practitioners, who saw themselves as physicians, surgeons and suppliers of medicines in one person, argued for a nation-wide system which could co-ordinate the efforts of all three sections of the medical profession.

Professional and trade institutions exist to promote the interests of their own members, however, which are not necessarily congruous with the interests of other parties or the public good. The Fellows of the Royal College of Physicians considered themselves to be the elite of the profession and, although sympathetic to the difficulties of the apothecaries-cum-general-practitioners, they were not prepared to sacrifice their own advantages to the interests of what they saw as a subservient sector of the medical system, rooted in trade. Or, to put it more bluntly, they could see no reason to encourage apothecaries to steal their business by becoming physicians to the lower classes even though those classes could never afford to consult a physician. The Royal College of Surgeons consisted of Fellows who lived in London and had profitable private practices and hospital interests and, like their physician colleagues, were unwilling to take responsibility for regulating provincial practitioners whose priorities were different from their own. Likewise, the Society of Apothecaries was a trading enterprise rather than a representative institution so its priority was its London trade, not the well-being of general practitioners. However, despite the apathy of the Colleges, the reluctance of the Society and the government's prior responsibility of winning the European war, the demand of the general practitioners for action was sympathetically heard by parliament and a bill was drafted.

The pressure for reform therefore came from general practitioners in London and the provinces who formed the great majority of the medical profession and had the most to gain from legislation, yet it was the Royal Colleges, which were only concerned with their own interests, who had the ear of government. Nevertheless, despite the lack of support from these influential bodies, an Act "for better regulating the Practice of Apothecaries throughout England and Wales" reached the Statute Book in 1815.[109] The principle objectives of the Act were to establish an educational system, to authorise an examination by which successful candidates were awarded licences to practice, and to suppress unlicensed competition to the profession throughout England and Wales. It did not change the Royal Colleges' right to regulate their own sections of the profession in London and it did not apply in Scotland. The Colleges were therefore not involved in implementing the Act which, in their view, only concerned an inferior form of medical practice, recently aggrandised from the apothecaries' trade. Responsibilities under the new Act were placed entirely on the London Society of Apothecaries, which it was not properly equipped to undertake because it was not an educational institution but a London-based trading company with little if any influence in the rest of England. And yet, despite all these disadvantages, the Apothecaries Act was the first legal measure to specify the educational requirements for the majority of the medical profession throughout England and Wales and was the beginning of a process that eventually united the profession. With this Act, the General Practitioner became a legally recognized being who was licensed to practice medicine, surgery and midwifery, as well as to dispense and sell medicines. It was a revolution which, though more peaceful than the industrial disturbances and less clamorous than the demand for electoral reform, was just as passionate because livelihoods were at stake. But there was a long way to go before the goal of a unified profession was achieved.

Under the Act, the Apothecaries' Society was required to

---

109 55 Geo.lll, c.194.

organise a qualifying examination, by which successful candidates were granted the 'Licence in Medicine and Surgery of the Society of Apothecaries' (LMSSA or more commonly LSA). Although the full title includes the words 'medicine' and 'surgery', pharmacy is only implied in 'Society of Apothecaries' and midwifery is not mentioned. The licence distinguished properly educated practitioners from the various pretenders to medical knowledge and skill. Preparation for the LSA examination therefore now required a longer and broader curriculum. So to demonstrate that they had completed the curriculum, candidates for the examination had to submit certificates of attendance at approved lectures and hospitals to the Court of Examiners. However, possession of a certificate was not necessarily evidence of having paid attention to the lecturer, or even of the student's presence in the lecture-room, so there was a ready market in certificates of dubious authenticity to make up for any failure of diligence on the part of the students. Although some provincial hospitals took a few students, anyone wanting to be a general practitioner was more or less obliged to attend the private London schools because they offered the broadest programmes of lectures and best clinical experience in England.

Edward finished his studies and left London in March 1814 just as legislation was being brought forward, so he was not affected by the new system. When news of the Apothecaries Act reached William and Edward in Coalbrookdale it must have seemed a radical measure because it changed the rules by which future general practitioners could enter practice. Edward was still only sixteen years old and would not complete his apprenticeship for another three years at least. When he did so, in 1818, the new law would require him to return to London for a longer time than he had anticipated and to take the LSA examination if he wanted to call himself a general practitioner. William had more or less promised that Edward could take another course in chemistry, but studying for the LSA would be a much more expensive proposition. Under the Act, apothecaries who had been practising before 1815 could continue to do so, but Edward had only been an apprentice, not a master, so could he legitimately continue if he did not take the LSA? Could they afford such a long period of study? Could William manage without Edward's help while he was away for two years? If not, could they afford to employ an assistant or another apprentice? This must have been a serious talking point for the family. Furthermore, their long-term future would depend on Edward's earning abilities which in turn depended on the prosperity of the struggling iron industry. Because of these uncertainties and because he could not sit the LSA until he was twenty-one years of age, Edward would have to contribute to the family livelihood in the shop for the next few years and bide his time until they could see what the future would bring. So he took up his responsibilities as intended, according to domestic demarcations agreed with his mother: the shop was to be his province while the house was hers, and though household deliveries would have to come through the shop he would manage it without interference from her.

In due course it became clear what Edward would have to do if he were to take his studies further. The Act did not define the curriculum for the LSA examination, but subject matter was inferred by the list of certificates of attendance at lectures and relevant experience which the candidates had to submit. The necessary certificates of attendance, which included the new subject of physiology, are shown in Table 5.1.

Table 5.1.
Requirements for entry to examination for LSA

Courses of Lectures	Number
Anatomy and Physiology	2
Theory and Practice of Medicine	2
Chemistry	1
Materia Medica (pharmacology)	1

Clinical Experience	
Attendance at the practice of a public hospital, infirmary or dispensary	6 months
Apprenticeship to an apothecary	5 years

All candidates must be competent in Latin

A 'course' of lectures lasted six months from October to March so it would take more than a year to complete two courses in Anatomy and Theory of Medicine, though Chemistry and *Materia Medica* could be taken at the same time as the others. William and Edward knew that 'Mr Brookes undertakes to teach anatomy in 3 months, for £50, board included'[110] but twice that time was now required for each course so would be more costly. In addition, after his theoretical studies Edward would have to do six months' clinical experience, so, including the summer vacation and the final examination, it would all take nearly two years. As well as the necessary fees he would have to find living costs so it was going to be expensive, perhaps two or three hundred pounds. As the income from the practice was probably no more than £200-300 pounds a year this would be a big drain on the family's finances. (In the light of changing money values, this was comparable to the

---

110 SA, 1987/56/15, Letter, William to Edward, 22 Feb 1814.

Twenty-First Century university fees of £8-9000 a year plus living costs, without loans being available). It was going to be several years before Edward could resume his studies and, in the meantime, much was happening in the world.

The revolutions that freed America from taxation and rule from London and ended the autocratic regime in France had profound effects on government of nations, though the price in war, cruelty and oppression had been high. In Britain, however, a degree of democracy had already been achieved by the Seventeenth Century Civil War and the struggle between Parliament and the restored Stuart monarchy, so pressure for further democratic reform had been contained while hostilities continued. But with reduction in external threat when peace returned, the clamour for greater representation of the people intensified. It was strengthened by the effect of industrialisation which changed the lives of those who worked in factories or were thrown out of work by the greater efficiency of mechanisation. By 1819, vigorous protests were being heard — which were peaceful until the infamous Peterloo massacre in Manchester. In and around Coalbrookdale the impoverished state of the iron industry provoked riots which were brutally suppressed.

Demands for reform and threat of rebellion were powerful, but discontent was not confined to the franchise nor to industry. By the Nineteenth Century it was Parliament and not the monarch who governed the land, though less than three percent of the male population had the right to vote and in only a few places did women have it. The House of Lords was entirely hereditary and therefore completely undemocratic. Worse still, many MPs represented so-called 'rotten boroughs' where a very few electors were prevailed upon to vote for the local landowner's or patron's nominees which, in retrospect, looks like corruption sanctioned by tradition and was certainly not democracy. An increasingly prosperous and educated population demanded a greater influence in the government of the country, not by violent revolution as in France, but by a fairer system for choosing its Members of Parliament. After 1815 and throughout the 1820s pressure for electoral reform increased until the Representation of the People and Municipal Corporations Acts of 1832 and 1835 were passed, though whether these really made much difference is debatable. The idea that people should have a say in their own government was gaining ground, eventually leading to the Chartist movement, the trade unions and large political parties. In the same way demands for better regulation of the medical profession were increasing from its own practitioners.

It soon became evident that the Apothecaries Act had not achieved the expectations of its protagonists, especially in the suppression of quackery. Though demands for reform originated in self-selected groups of ordinary practitioners, these were largely ignored because the Royal Colleges and the Society of Apothecaries were not representative bodies. Representation of opinion among general practitioners therefore mirrored the old parliamentary electoral system: political influence was confined to the oligarchic and self-interested groups which, like pocket boroughs, did not represent the views of the majority of the 'common people', ie the thousands of general practitioners. The Colleges refused to undertake regulation of this new kind of doctor that had recently appeared with popular approval in a free market, and the Society of Apothecaries was failing in its responsibility to do so. As the years went by the failings of the Act became apparent and, by the 1830s, these three bodies were challenged by William Farr, an exact contemporary of Edward's. He described them in his short-lived journal, *British Annals of Medicine,* as:

> ... unreformed medical corporations, floating down from antiquity like icebergs, freezing and darkly frowning on the life and freedom of these sunnier times. Some hundred physicians and 21 London surgeons and a

trading band of Apothecaries ... rule in unrestrained licence over all the physicians, surgeons and general practitioners of the empire.[111]

Farr may have been a little fanciful in his choice of metaphor, but he was in tune with demands for a better system of representation that were soon to be heard throughout the profession in parallel with reformist activity in the country at large. It would take another forty years for a better, though not perfect, system to be devised.

While these sentiments were being voiced in England, an entirely peaceful medical revolution occurred in France. In many countries, including Britain, the old 'constitutional' or 'humoral' ideas about the causes of disease were being replaced by theories that associated illnesses with specific disorders of internal organs such as the heart, lungs or kidneys. In gathering information in patients with respiratory and heart diseases, it had become common practice for doctors to listen to the heart beating and the air moving in and out of the lungs by placing an ear on the patient's chest. One day in 1816, twenty-seven-year-old René Laennec, a physician at the Hôpital Necker in Paris, was confronted with a problem in the form of a young woman whom he described as having such 'a great degree of fatness' as to muffle the sounds of breathing. Whether from delicate consideration of her age and sex or his own reluctance, for we know nothing of his patient's cleanliness, he was not inclined to place his ear on her chest and, in looking for an alternative, had an inspiration. He knew that sound is conducted better in solid material than air, so he rolled up a sheaf of papers into a stout tube and placed one end of this on her chest and put his ear to the other. He was delighted to discover that he could hear the sounds of his patient's breathing and the beating of her heart more clearly than

---

111 Farr, W., Progress of the medical profession — obstructions in its way, *British Annals of Medicine,* 19 May 1837.

by the usual method.[112] He had invented the stethoscope.[113]

It was four years before Laennec published his discovery and many more before doctors adopted the stethoscope in practice, though it is now a kind of badge of office. Yet it was a major step in demonstrating the state of the lungs and heart and it encouraged doctors to find ways to examine other internal organs. In the subsequent two hundred years, all sorts of 'scope' instruments have been devised to peer into ears, eyes, throats and other less alluring parts of the human body. Diagnosis by recognition of internal signs had arrived and it would have profound implications for medical education and practice. Contemporaries of Edward, and his young brother Benjamin when it came to his turn, would be among the first to adopt these techniques — if they were progressive enough to do so.

---

112   Porter, R, *The Greatest Benefit to Mankind; a medical history of humanity from antiquity to the present.* London, Fontana Press, 1997, pp 308-9.

113   From the Greek στῆϑος chest + σκοπ-εῖν to look at, observe. OED on-line edition, 3 Mar 2013

Plates

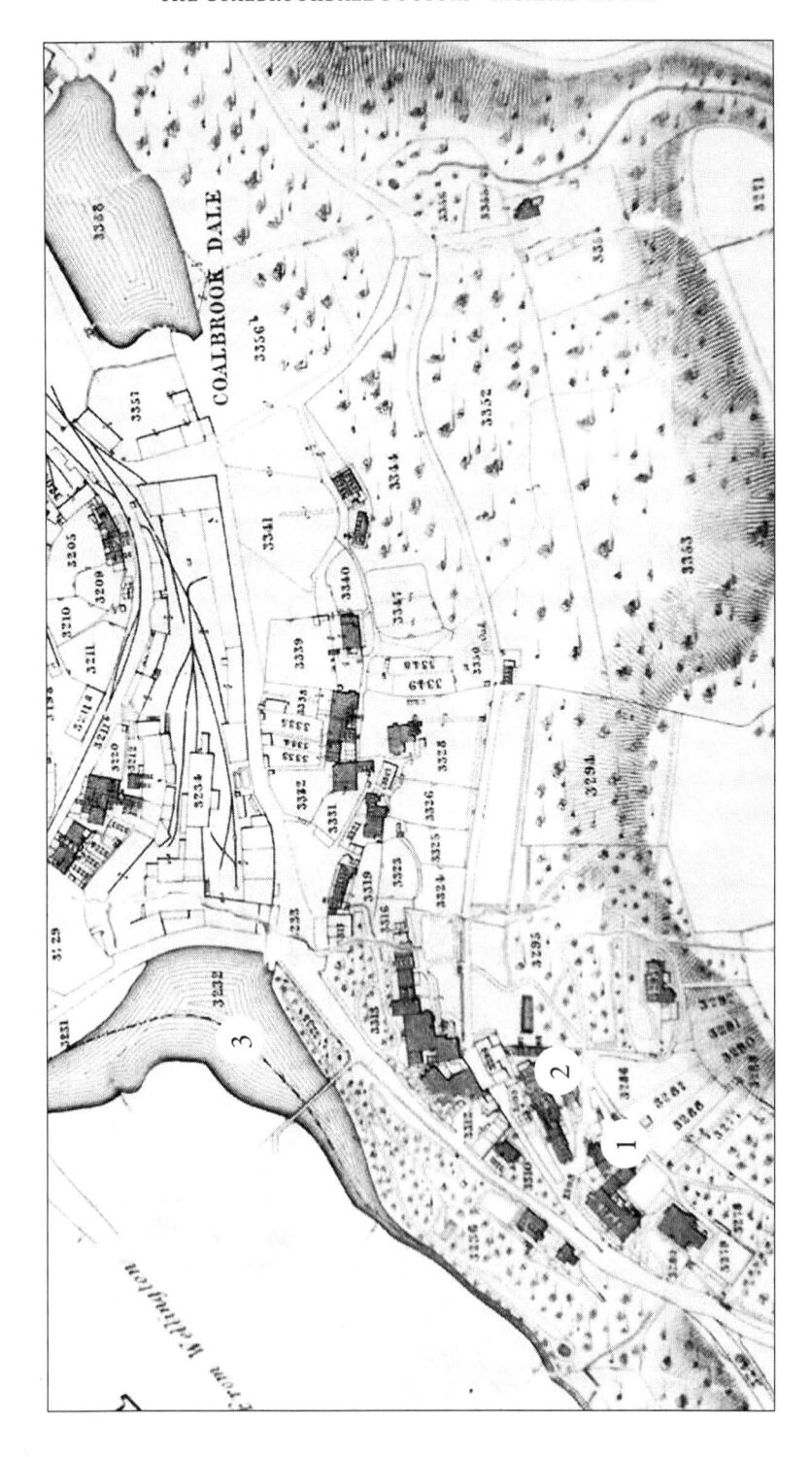
COALBROOK DALE
1
2
3

PLATES

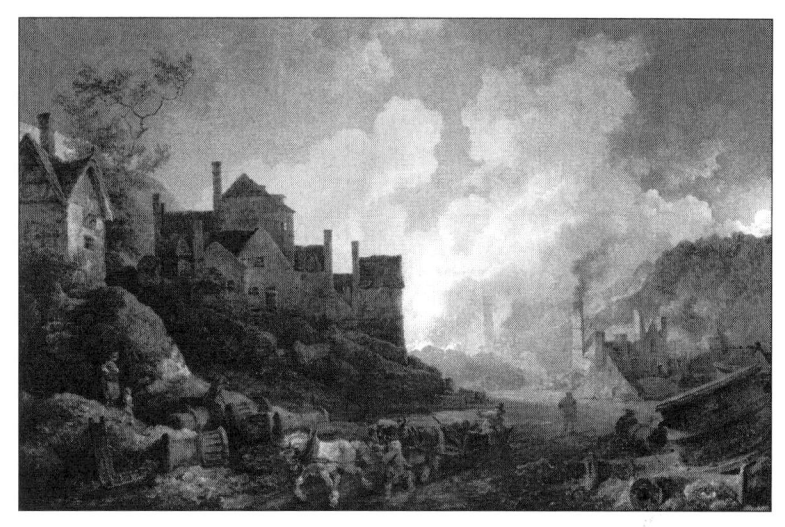

2. *Coalbrookdale at Night*, by Philip James de Loutherburg, 1801,
Science Museum, London.
A fiery glow illuminates the sky of innumerable furnaces, day and night.
In the foreground lie heaps of iron castings and industrial detritus.

1. Opposite:
Map of Coalbrookdale, from Tithe Map 1849, Shropshire Archives.
Rose Hill (1), Teakettle Row (2) and the Upper Furnace Pool (3) are indicated.

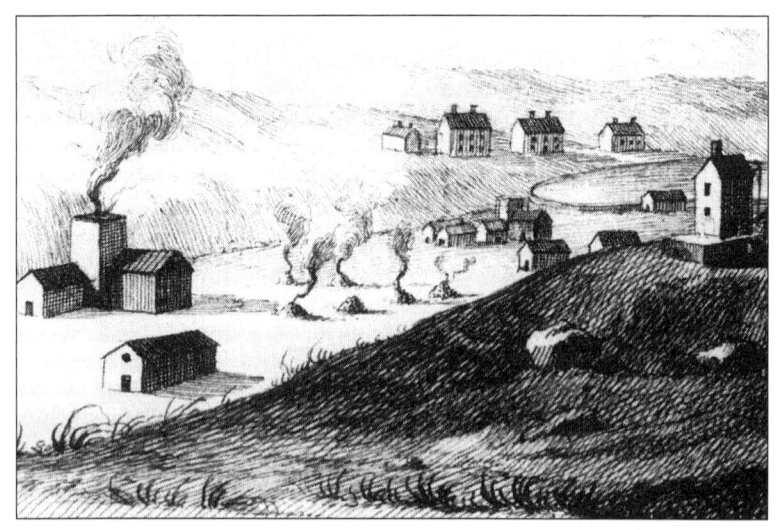

3. *Coalbrookdale Works, Fire Engine and Mill-pond, from R. R. Angerstein's Travel Diary, 1753-1755: Industry in England and Wales from a Swedish perspective*, Ironbridge Gorge Museum Trust Collection.

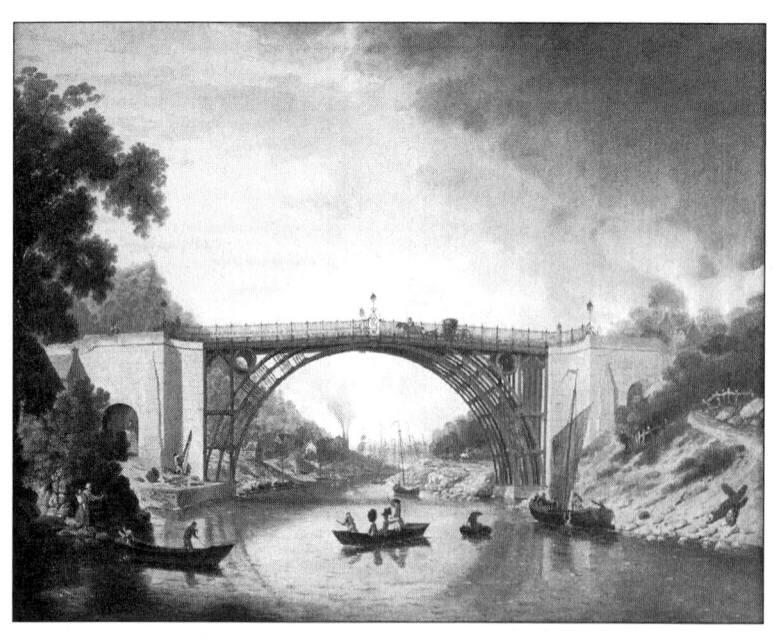

4. *The Iron Bridge*, by William Williams, 1779, Ironbridge Gorge Museum Trust Collection. Benjamin Wright probably saw the bridge being built.

PLATES

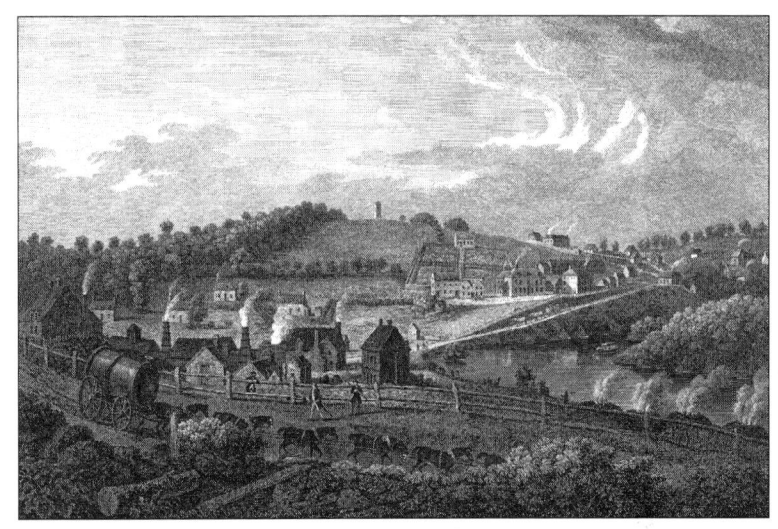

5. *A View of the Upper Works at Coalbrookdale*, by François Vivares, 1758, Ironbridge Gorge Museum Trust Collection.
The Upper Works are in the foreground, with the Ironmasters houses visible beyond the Upper Furnace Pool. Rose Hill is only sketchily shown. The smoking heaps beside the pool consist of coal being converted to coke.

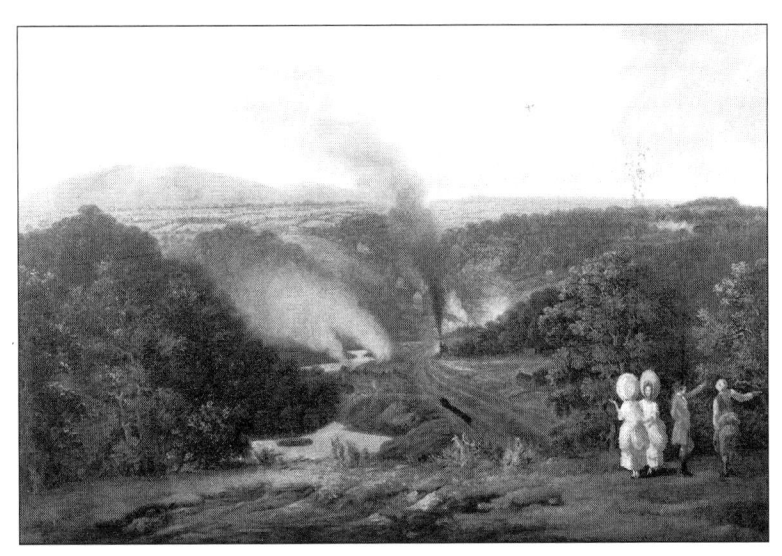

6. *An afternoon view of Coalbrookdale*, by William Williams, 1771, Shropshire Council, Shropshire Museum.
The Wrekin can be seen in the distance, with Rose Hill and the Darby houses in the centre, almost obscured by 'fuliginous' chimneys which pollute the otherwise sylvan Dale. (cf Anna Seward's poem *Coalbrookdale*).

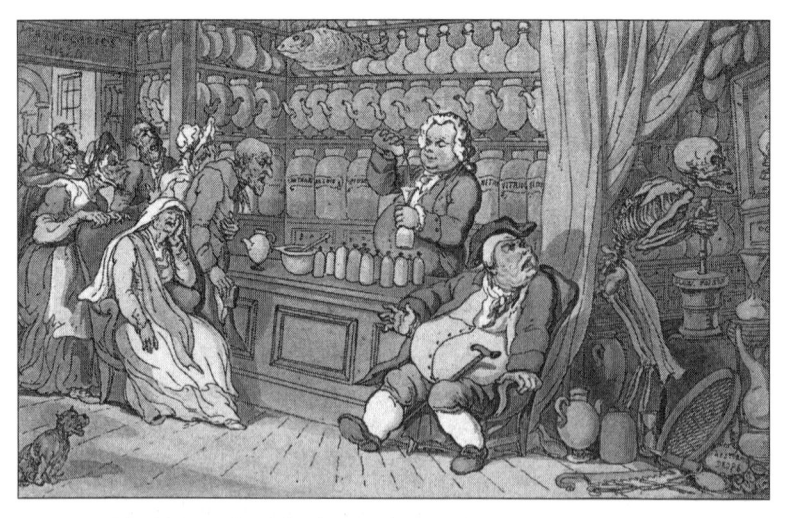

7. *The Dance of Death: the Apothecary,* by T. Rowlandson, 1816, Wellcome Library, London.

The caricature shows an apothecary's shop with a queue of sick people awaiting their turns, while behind a curtain a skeletal apprentice prepares stock medicines. It is to be hoped that the Edwards's shop was more welcoming than this one.

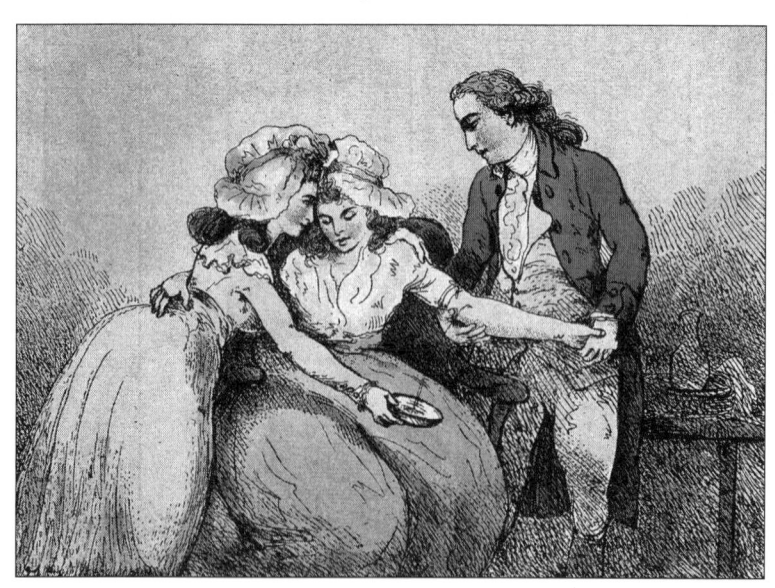

8. *A surgeon bleeding the arm of a young woman,* by T. Rowlandson, 1784, Wellcome Library, London.

Bleeding by opening a vein was a common treatment for many illnesses in the Eighteenth and early Nineteenth Centuries.

PLATES

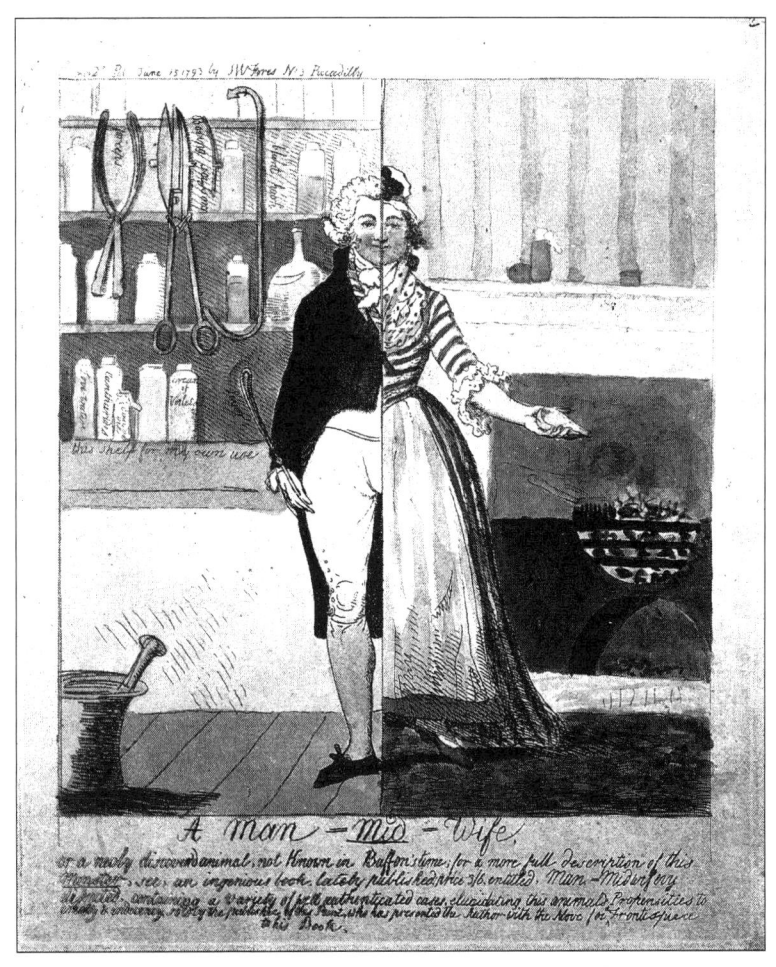

9. *A Man-Mid-Wife, a newly discovered animal not known before,* by Isaac Cruikshank, 1793, Wellcome Library, London.
The practice of midwifery by male surgeons was a new idea in the Eighteenth Century. The drawing shows a split figure, left side female, right side male.

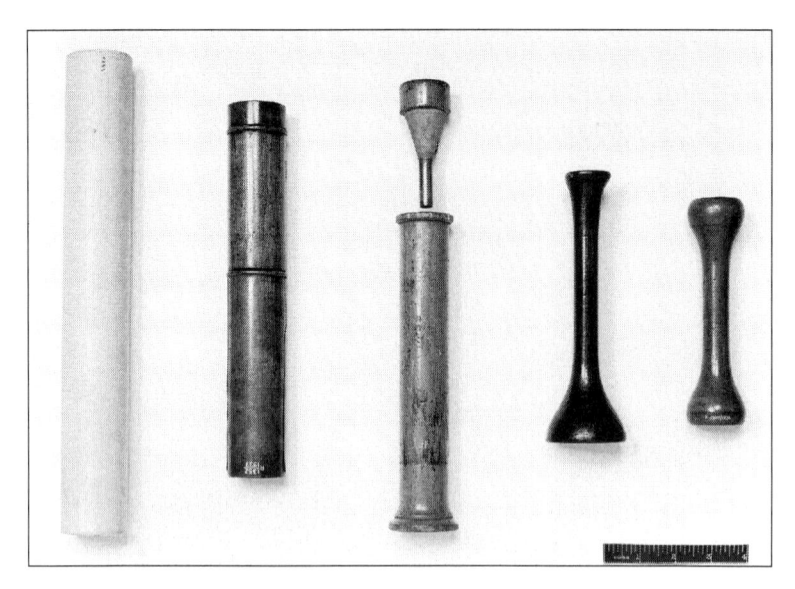

10. *A collection of Laennec's stethoscopes*, early 19th Century, Wellcome Library, London.
Laennec invented the stethoscope in 1816, and published his invention and its uses in in 1819.

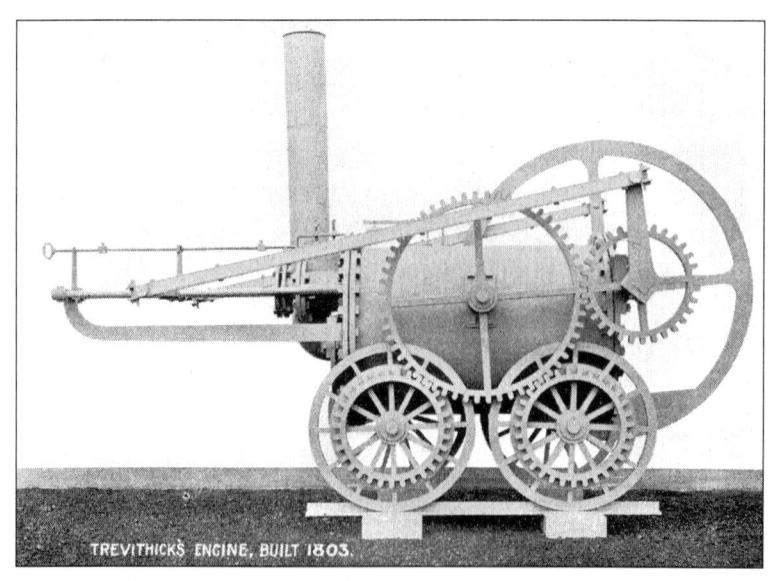

11. *Reconstruction of Trevithick's steam locomotive*, built in 1803, Ironbridge Gorge Museum Trust Collection.
Trevithick's first mobile steam engine was built in Cornwall but it was for for use on roads. This was the first locomotive to run on rails.

PLATES

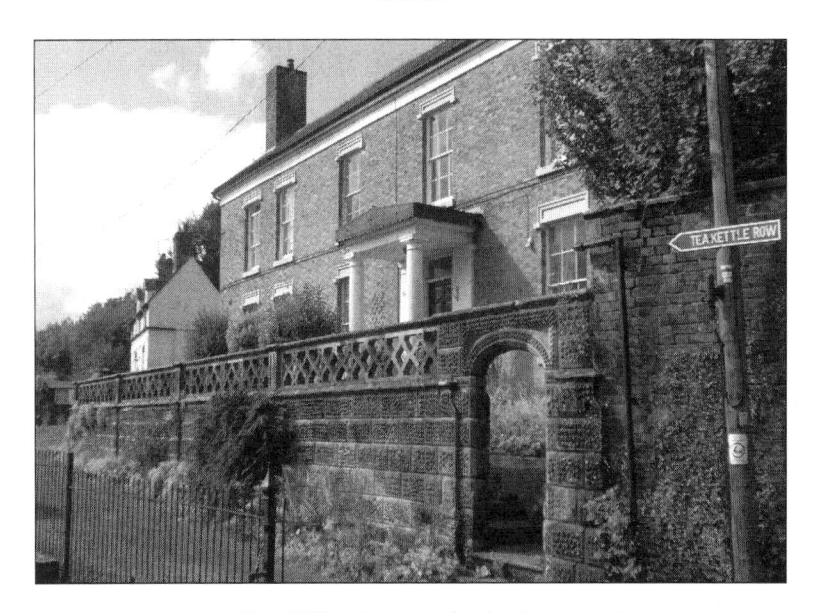

12. *Rose Hill in 2014*, author's photograph.

Chapter 6

Edward in London

After his return to Coalbrookdale in 1814, Edward finished his apprenticeship and became one of the Coalbrookdale doctors. Like many of his contemporaries, however, he still cherished a desire to further his education so he returned to London in October 1821 at the age of twenty-two. Even six years after the Apothecaries Act, its significance for the future of medical practice had still not been fully realised and there was some doubt whether Edward should take the examination for the LSA. It would certainly make him a fully qualified general practitioner, but it would require nearly two years of study which would be very expensive and take him away from the business for much of that time.

In the meantime much had been happening both in the Edwards family and in the wider world. In 1818 Richard was seventeen years old and, if his previously half-hearted interest in the business had been revived, he could have been apprenticed to his father. Certainly there were plans for him to go to London to stay with his uncle Richard.[114] He was to travel in one of the new horse-drawn 'fly-boats' on the river and canal system because they were cheaper and far more comfortable than the rattling stage coaches (by 1821 it was possible, for example, to go from Stourport to Gloucester on a Steam Packet carrying five hundred passengers and return the same day, a distance of eighty-six miles.[115]) But plans for Richard's future bore no fruit because by the end of 1821 he was dead. He was buried in the Quaker burial ground near his grandfather Benjamin who, in earlier years, had also suffered

---

114 SA, 1986/56/1, Letter, Richard Edwards (senior) to William Edwards (senior), 23 Jul 1818.

115 *Shrewsbury Chronicle*, 7 Sep 1821.

an untimely death. Richard's younger brother, fifteen-year-old William, was a boarder at Adams grammar school in Newport. He wrote to Edward thanking him for sending some apples, though it had not been a fruitful year in the garden, and telling him about his school work: in class he was reading Cicero and the third book of Virgil in Latin, and out of school he had begun to read Homer.[116] He asked Edward to tell his sister Anna Maria that he would write to her 'very soon' and would be glad to see her and perhaps Fanny or Betsey if they came to Newport. Such homely touches permeate the surviving correspondence of this close and friendly family.

Beyond the family and their neighbours in the Dale, the country was troubled by the aftermath of war. A fortunate few prospered from the more efficient manufacturing brought about by new machinery in large factories, from better transport and flourishing enterprises in the colonies — where slaves continued to work until 1833 even though the trading in slaves had been illegal since 1807. In Britain, workers in factories and mines felt ever more oppressed by the widespread unemployment and reduction of the wages of those still in work. The Corn Laws, intended to maintain the profits of landowners and growers in the face of competition from cheaper imports, caused a critical rise in the price of food and near-starvation for the poorest people from which Coalbrookdale and its neighbourhood were not spared. By 1818, some of the blast furnaces in the Dale as well as another twenty-four furnaces in other parts of Shropshire had ceased operation. In 1817, the workers in Coalbrookdale went on strike to support Black Country colleagues whose jobs were threatened.[117] The distress from such a severe economic decline was made worse by a disastrous harvest.[118] Before the introduction of the modern system

---

116 SA, 1986/56/20, Letter, William (junior) to Edward, Sep 1820.

117 Trinder, B., *The Industrial Revolution in Shropshire*, p. 231.

118 Raistrick, A., *Dynasty of Ironfounders: the Darbys of Coalbrookdale*, p 289-90.

of social security, starving families depended on the meagre support of their parishes or, if they were fortunate, on the largesse of their employers. Parishes could give small money doles for food or, in the last resort, take individuals or whole families into the poor houses, though in Madeley at this time they were in a state of neglect. William was medical officer to the parish [119] and, if these unfortunate people fell seriously ill, the burden of treating them fell to him, though with such scanty payment for doing so that his own financial state must have suffered too.

In the political field, the drive for representation in government gathered momentum. A population without the means of expressing their views to those in authority is powerless except by taking to the streets for public demonstration of their grievances. One such event was the notorious Peterloo Massacre in Manchester in August 1819. Textile workers there had suffered a drastic reduction of wages from fifteen to five shillings a week, at the same time as the cost of food was rising sharply. The Manchester Patriotic Union, a responsible organisation seeking political reform, feared that there would be insurrection if grievances were not brought to the attention of those who had the power to remedy them and planned a meeting in a large open space called St Peter's Fields. The magistrates banned it because they feared it would lead to violent disorder, but the defiant organisers simply postponed it for a week. Unable to prevent the meeting, the magistrates summoned over one thousand troops, consisting of 120 cavalrymen, a troop with two six-pounder field guns, and a large number of armed but ill-trained militia men. The magistrates were watching from a nearby house and, when they saw vigorous confrontations beginning between demonstrators and troops, they ordered the soldiers to disperse the crowds at bayonet point. When this failed because the escape route was blocked, the troops opened fire. Seven men and four women were

---

119 Smith, L., Refuges of last Resort, *Transactions of the Shropshire Archaeological and Historical Society*, Vol. LXXXII, 2007, p 58.

killed, and more than six hundred others were injured. Rioting and shooting continued for the rest of day and even spread to Oldham a few miles away where another man was killed.

These drastic events took place far from the Edwards family and the people of Coalbrookdale, but the economic depression affected the Shropshire coalfield as much as anywhere, so work was scarce and wages low. Only five months after the Peterloo massacre some Shropshire ironmasters announced that wages would be further reduced which provoked anger that erupted into violence. On 31 January 1820, five hundred men and women (who were as angry as their men-folk) assembled at the spoil heaps at the Old Park Works, the so-called 'Cinder Hills'. News of the gathering spread and the crowd swelled to over three thousand.[120] Gangs of angry men and women marched from one works to another, removing the plugs from the boilers to let out the steam and drain the water, thereby halting production. They eventually returned to Old Park where they were confronted by a magistrate, Mr Cludde, seated in his carriage surrounded by constables, and were persuaded to go home peacefully. The next day they assembled again and breaking into groups rampaged about the various works at Dawley Castle, Stirchley, Lawley Bank and Coalbrookdale with riotous behaviour, wielding sticks, throwing stones and causing further damage. They returned to the vantage point of the Cinder Hills where they were confronted by five magistrates supported by a troop of cavalry. One of the magistrates, Mr Thomas Eyton, read the Riot Act which was a formal announcement that punitive action would be taken if the crowd did not disperse within one hour. Although Eyton's voice could hardly be heard over the shouting, the reading of the Riot Act did produce a temporary calm, but the angry crowd failed to melt away as instructed and two men were arrested. As they were being marched off surrounded by the cavalry, a barrage of stones and cinders was hurled at the escort and, in the confusion, the prisoners escaped. The

---

120 *Salopian Journal*, 28 Mar. 1820, Trial of the Colliers.

magistrates decided that this was a 'tumultuous and illegal assembly' and this authorised Eyton to order the troops to open fire. Two men were killed and another, Thomas Palin, was wounded.[121] Seven men were arrested, including Palin who was, however, allowed to have his wounds dressed by a surgeon, Uriel Cooper from Donnington. They were all charged with riotous assembly and tried a month later in Shrewsbury where evidence of doubtful quality was heard, including that of a twelve-year-old boy. In summing up, the judge conceded that men 'had a right to ask respectfully for an advance of wages, and could leave if they were not satisfied with the answer given' (though he did not suggest how they might find other work if they did leave). But, he said, destruction of their master's property was not only illegal but would prevent further employment for everyone. The jury took 'only a few minutes' to return a verdict of Guilty, at which the judge advised the seven men 'to seek God's redemption in the time left to them in this life' and sentenced them all to hang.

The riots must have been a frightening time for everyone, including the Edwards family. William and Edward were probably called upon to treat people wounded in the scuffles because as well as those injured by shooting there would have been many others who were hit by flying stones, crushed by cudgels or knocked down in the confusion. The Edwards family and their neighbours must have feared for their safety because their house was only a few hundred yards from the works where these angry protests were happening, and they were very close to the homes of the Darby family. It was not unknown for leading citizens and their houses to be attacked: not long before this an angry mob had burned Joseph Priestley's house in Birmingham because of his sympathies with the French revolution. The harsh judgement of the court after the Cinder Hill riots made further public demonstration of discontent too risky and, though outbreaks of anger at the low wages and harsh conditions erupted from time to time in Coalbrookdale

---

121 Trinder, B., *The Industrial Revolution in Shropshire*, p. 232.

and elsewhere, none were as bad as those of 1820. The grievances of labouring men and women were eventually taken up by the Chartist and trades-union movements, as well as by philanthropic individuals, and in due course improvements in pay and working conditions were achieved through the Factory Acts and other legislation. But it was a long road.

The national economy remained depressed and the future of the Coalbrookdale Company uncertain. A visitor to the works in 1821 noted that the place 'appeared to be much neglected'.[122] If the Edwards' medical business was to prosper in the economic depression, the questions about Edward's education had to be resolved: should he return to London for further study, and if so should he take the LSA which would take up to two years? Would there be enough work for both him and his father in the present state of affairs? Should he therefore look for work elsewhere? It was agreed that, despite the uncertainties, Edward should return to London for further study but a decision on the examination was deferred. In October 1821 he went to London to start a course of lectures, lodging with Mr Blackley in Dean Street, Soho.[123] His mother, Elizabeth, wrote to him with all the gossip of the Dale expressed in her usual lugubrious style. She had been in a 'poor state of health' since Edward had been there last and, though she was feeling better, the pain in her side remained although 'through mercy' she was able to look after her family. She passed on a message from six-year-old Benjamin to say that he had 'been a good boy two mornings, and [Edward] must buy him a two-shilling band of music' — an early indication of his musical interest and perhaps of a deviant tendency. William had been 'pretty much engaged in the day time' so he tended to fall asleep in the evenings through fatigue. Edward's uncle, Peter Wright, had 'had a violent quarrel over [some] game' with his brother-

---

122 Raistrick, A., *Dynasty of Ironfounders: the Darbys of Coalbrookdale*, p 246.

123 SA, 1957/56/17, Letter, Elizabeth to Edward, Jan 1822.

in-law Yate who had 'sent him a challenge', that is to say summons to a duel, but fortunately the quarrel was settled without violence.

Elizabeth gave news of some of Williams patients. There had been 'two very aweful [sic] instances of the uncertainties of life':

> John Richard's Wife who lived at Lamhole went past here last night much as usual and died at two this morning. Captain Donnel of Madeley was at market on Friday and died on Wednesday following.

Concerning her relatives, 'Mr G. Morgan has been very ill with a Rheumatick complaint', though on the bright side Mr W. Morgan was supplying 'excellent bread at a good price'. Ever careful for the safety of her son, she concluded with this advice:

> I hope you will keep out of publick places till your next journey [to return home]. I also wish to caution you against going in the steam boats there has been a very bad accident happened, we saw an account of it in the Shrewsbury paper.

Edward had evidently raised the matter of the LSA again, for she wrote:

> If you think it is absolutely necessary to take the diploma I think you had better write to your father respecting it, he wants you at home very much and hopes you will come home as soon as you possibly can.

Elizabeth's next letter opened with a sigh of relief. She had been expecting news of Edward for a long time, and inevitably feared it would be bad. But he was safe after all. She wrote:

> [I am] very thankful to hear you are well, I sincerely hope [that] your going to church in future will not be out of mere curiosity but to return thanks to your heavenly father who has so mercifully preserved you when you have seen your fellow pupils so awefully visited, into his hands I have committed you humbly trusting that he will preserve you from the dangers, snares and temptations that you are exposed to.

What can have happened to his fellow students? Had they been robbed, or had they fallen through the ice on the Thames? Were they in debt from gambling? Or had they caught some fatal disease from their patients? It remains a mystery.

Later Elizabeth gave more news of the business, which was not good. William was 'losing a great number of Midwifery cases' which were 'too numerous to mention', perhaps because of an outbreak of puerperal fever, that mysterious disease that we now know (but they did not) is caused by the same germ as that which causes sore throats and scarlet fever. Midwifery had been worrying other doctors in the area, too. She reported that Mr Procter had called William to a dangerous case, though the 'patient is likely to do well'. As well as routine medical cases, Edward had been doing some of the midwifery and was popular with expectant mothers so his return to London was a disappointment to his patients. Elizabeth wrote: 'there are some that want you at home very badly ... we have many enquiries after you wishing you a speedy and safe return especially the Ladyes [sic]'. Edward's skill as a man-midwife may have been noteworthy, but even the best man-midwife might not have been able to prevent tragic loss of life from the hazards of childbirth without the techniques that are now available. For example:

> Mrs Cookson is safely put to bed after having a very dangerous time and a dead child...

> Your father lost another case last night it was William Wilson's wife at Croppings...

> Poor Mrs Richards is very unwell she has never recovered from her confinement. Your father thinks she is consumptive...

Or was Mrs Richards suffering from the so-far unrecognised post-natal depression?

Then comes another warning of moral danger that Elizabeth feared her son would be exposed to. She had been reading a 'very nice book' that was 'no fiction' about a seriously-minded young man who went to work in London despite his mother's fears that he would be corrupted there. In due course the lad met with 'improper company and suffered severely'. Careful not to loosen the apron-strings too much, Elizabeth advised her twenty-three-year-old son to be 'very cautious in forming acquaintances, it is better to be alone than in bad company'. The question of the LSA rumbled on: his father still thought he would 'do very well without taking the diploma [because] it is only an honorary form', though it probably did not seem like that to the candidates for examination. As a man of the Eighteenth Century, William was unable to foresee the inevitable changes that were coming to the medical profession but Edward, whose future was in the Nineteenth, needed the education and qualifications that would fit him to be a doctor in the scientific age that was then dawning.

Edward was determined to take the examination, but needed his father's agreement because only he could supply the necessary certificate of apprenticeship. It took a long time to get William's consent. No letter from William discussing the matter survives but, when the decision was finally made, Edward's sister Betsey wrote: 'I think it is requisite that you should pass and you are quite right in clearing it, the certificate shall be procured and sent in time for you'.[124] Betsey sent news of the

---

124 SA, 1987/56/19, Letter, Betsey to Edward.

family business in the same letter — it was very demanding for her father. For example, one day he returned from a long journey of home visits to find a 'shopful' of people but was immediately called out to another emergency. An elderly woman, Mrs Richards, had fallen over an old carpet and broken her thigh. William did what was possible at that time but her husband, whom Betsey referred to as 'an old mouse', was not satisfied and demanded a second opinion from his own doctor, Mr Gwynne. William saw no need for this and declined to arrange it. The 'old mouse' heaped insults upon William though Betsey did not pass on the phrases he used, perhaps to the disappointment of curious readers. She turned to pleasanter topics: the bees were doing well; their musical cousin Sarah Wright had been studying the organ in Shrewsbury and hoped to be appointed organist at a Broseley church; and 'Little Ben' said 'he hopes you will buy him a fiddle and a gun'.

With his father's approval now obtained, Edward applied to take the examination in May 1824. More than two years had gone by since he had returned to London which was far longer than William had anticipated, though, because the courses only ran from October to April, Edward probably returned to the business during the long summer vacations. While he was away he was badly missed by patients and family because, not only was he a popular doctor and much in demand for his abilities as a man-midwife, but he had been a severe drain on the family's resources. He must have been an ardent student because he had taken three courses more than the rules required: an extra course in each of Anatomy and Physiology, Chemistry and *Materia Medica*, as well as the mandatory two of Theory and Practice of Medicine, two of Chemistry and six months clinical work, which he did at the Western General Dispensary.[125]

---

125   Payne, J., Archivist at the Society of Apothecaries, personal communication. The record shows that Edward had taken one more course in each of Anatomy and Physiology, Chemistry and *Materia Medica* than the regulations required. He seems to have been an enthusiastic student.

By the standards of the time the LSA was a great educational advance because it was the first assessment of medical competence by public examination to be introduced and it must have seemed a stiff challenge to the candidates, of whom there was no shortage. It probably challenged students to study thoroughly for fear of being found wanting but, if judged by modern methods of assessment, it was not a very searching test. It only consisted of a few minutes oral examination by one person and could not have tested their knowledge in any depth. The Apothecaries Society, which was not an academic institution, had had the new examination thrust upon it by parliament despite having no experience of organising such a thing. The Society was managed by the Governor and a Court of Assistants whose members were chosen according to seniority. Conduct of the examination was delegated to the twelve most senior members of the Court of Assistants, called the Court of Examiners, in other words the oldest members of the Society whose knowledge was likely to be seriously out of date in this period of rapid scientific progress. Whatever its defects, successful candidates were licensed to practise and entitled to call themselves 'physician and surgeon' and for the first time they could be distinguished from untrained pretenders to those skills.

The Court of Examiners met weekly on Thursdays. Candidates had to give written notice of their intention to be examined on or before the Monday of the week in which they wished to be examined and to attend at Apothecaries' Hall on the following Thursday at 'half-past one o'clock'. On arrival they had to present the required certificates to the Society's Beadle and were warned that attempts to influence him by crossing his palm with silver were not to be tolerated:

> It is expressly ordered that no gratuity may be received by any officer from any person applying for information relative to the business of the Court of Examiners'.

Topics which might be covered included: the translation from the Latin of parts of the *Pharmacopoeia Londonensis* and a selection of physicians' prescriptions; pharmaceutical chemistry; and *Materia Medica*. There was no attempt to assess clinical knowledge.

Edward was examined by Mr Tegart at Apothecaries' Hall on 13th May 1824 and was 'approved'. News of his success reached Coalbrookdale on May 15th, only two days later, and his sister Fanny wrote to him immediately with the family's congratulations.[126] Edward was not allowed to revel in his success with his friends for long because William was feeling the strain of running the business on his own and wanted him to return at once. Fanny wrote:

> We are all very gratified to hear you had passed Apothecaries Hall, and that your mind is made easy on that account. It is my mother's particular desire that I write by return of Post, to say how badly you are wanted, particularly yesterday, my Father had been a long journey and had just finished his dinner, when a messenger came to fetch him to a bad case at Little Wenlock, he sent to Broseley for Mr Gwynn but he not being at home Mr Thursfield went. Till then we had been tolerably well with the exception of two midwifery cases which were lost, and we know not how many more might have been saved if you had been at home ... my father has been as well as usual and has borne the fatigue of the journeys surprisingly. My mother is much better but she is not willing to own it.

Having passed on the message that Edward was so badly needed at home, Fanny, now sixteen, expressed her envy of his adventures in London and indulged in a little adolescent day-dreaming:

---

126 SA, 1987/56/22, Letter, Fanny to Edward.

I should very much like to go with you to see the Theatres but as to fine Cloathes I have no particular desire for any of them unless I was there myself with the one thing needful [money] but I believe I must rest contentedly at home. I have nothing more to say except we all join in love

    Believe me my dear Edward

    Your Affectt. Sister, Fanny

    PS. I am almost ashamed to send this scrawl, but I hope you will excuse it.

It was the lot of women to run the home while men ran the world.

Edward, now qualified as 'physician, surgeon and apothecary', returned to Coalbrookdale to take up the burden of the business including his former duties in the shop and a share of the journeys. There is no record of events in the business or at Rose Hill for the next few years because the correspondence ceased on Edward's return. The household was still busy however because, by 1824, there were six of the family at home — William and Elizabeth, Betsey, Edward, Fanny and Anna Maria — plus the servants. Young Benjamin would also have been at home in the holidays from his boarding school, though the whereabouts of William, now nineteen, are unknown.

Next news of the family comes in a letter in April 1828 from eighteen-year-old Anna Maria to twelve-year-old Benjamin at John Woods School at Shifnal.[127] The good news was that she hoped to be able to visit him soon (he was only ten miles away but she would probably have to walk); the bad news was that Edward had heard that Benjamin was 'in the habit of betting', and Anna Maria passed on his hope that 'he may never hear of it again as it is a very bad practice'. Edward also expected that Benjamin could repeat the *1st Book of Homer*,

---

127 SA, 1987/56/33, Letter, Fanny to William and Benjamin.

one of the classical authors who featured largely in their education. Anna Maria said her mother was sorry she had not sent him a cake which was because there was more bad news — Fanny was ill:

> You will be very sorry when I tell you how dangerously ill my Sister Fanny has been, I have no doubt you expected she was quite recovered from a slight indisposition she had when you left home but it degenerated into Typhus Fever a complaint very prevalent at present.

That dread disease had raised its ugly head again, possibly brought home by her father from one of his patients. The reader will recall that Benjamin Wright had suffered a similar illness in 1794, when Rebecca Darby had noted that he had 'laboured under great disposition' (though somehow 'disposition' had now become '*in*disposition'). If they now feared for Fanny's life they had good reason to do so because typhus was a killer. At that time, more than 12,000 of the twelve million people in England and Wales died of it every year.[128] A contemporary text book describes the symptoms of 'languor, chilliness and depressed spirits, with sighing and oppression of the breathing; pain in the head; confusion of thought; vomiting; pulse quick and weak; the countenance is expressive of anxiety.' After two weeks there would be a 'crisis' with rigors, sweating and collapse, when the patient might die. Fanny would have been treated with emetics to 'remove congestion and equalize the circulation' and would have been kept lying flat. She would have had her head shaved, blisters applied to the back of the neck and been bled, either by opening a vein in the arm or by applying eight or ten leeches to the temples.[129] She was fortunate to survive though

---

128 Charlton, J. and Murphy, M., *The Health of Adult Britain, 1841-1994*, London, The Stationery Office, 1997, p. 32.

129 Steggall, J., *A manual for students preparing for examination at Apothecaries Hall or other medical examinations*, London, John Churchill, 1838, p 465.

the treatment cannot now be said to have cured her. Her recovery would have been uncertain and prolonged and her family would have feared for her life.

In September 1828, there was worse: William died. He was only fifty-six years old. Had the strain of the business been too much for him? Had he caught pneumonia after being drenched on one of those long journeys to see patients? Or, like his daughter Fanny and possibly his predecessor Benjamin, had he succumbed to the ever-prevalent typhus? The record of William's death was in a letter to Edward from his uncle Richard.[130] He began with his regret at 'receiving the intelligence of this melancholy event', and was sorry he was unable to travel to Coalbrookdale for his brother's funeral because it would be too long a journey for him. He was interested to know 'in what circumstances he has left his family and what disposition he has made of his property', by which he means his share of the inheritance of their father's estate in Norfolk. There had evidently been some doubt about this because Richard says that William had been 'chosen out of' that property, as well as another in Denver, by 'impossible' wills that had been 'cooked up' by witnesses who had been 'procured for a trifle'.

William's untimely death must have been a terrible shock to the family, especially if it was sudden. As a life-long and devout Anglican, albeit with Quaker sympathies, he was interred at Malinslee church. We can picture the scene at his funeral: the family, clad in black and the ladies veiled, stand beside the open grave to see the coffin lowered into the cold earth. Grief chills their souls as the first grey mists of autumn chill their bodies. Many others, who have known him for years as their friend, neighbour or doctor, gather round them to share their grief and their loss.

Edward was now the only doctor in the practice and would have to shoulder the whole burden of it himself. He would have to answer to both shop and visiting and, though there were friendly relations with

---

130 SA, 1987/56/25, Letter, Richard Edwards (senior) to Edward.

colleagues to help with difficult cases, patients would go elsewhere if they could not get the attention they sought in the competitive market for medical services. At the age of twenty-nine Edward was now the family's breadwinner, responsible for the livelihood of his mother, three sisters and his young brother Benjamin. William junior was twenty-four and presumably earning his living elsewhere, which may have been as a schoolmaster at Shifnal.[131] For Elizabeth, her husband's death was a tragedy and perhaps a disaster because she, seemingly, was not the most resilient of characters. For Fanny, who had largely recovered from her illness, the grief of losing her father would surely have delayed her convalescence. As for thirteen-year-old Benjamin, Edward clearly had firm views on his young brother's behaviour, at least as far as betting was concerned, and, as head of the family, he was now responsible for his brother's welfare. This was a role which he was to take seriously in years to come when Benjamin went to London and met those temptations which had frightened his mother so much when Edward had been there years before.

To the relief of everyone, Fanny slowly recovered from the illness that had been such a worry, but more bad news awaited them: in February 1829 young William died. He was only twenty four and the cause of his death is unknown. Some sense of the family's shock is recorded in a letter to Edward from Elizabeth's brother Benjamin Wright. His thoughts and feelings, and probably those of the whole family, are best expressed in his own words:[132]

> I have only this day received yours of the 5th inst containing the melancholy information of the death of your Brother William. I assure you Edward I most deeply

---

131 SA, 1987/56/12, Letter, Anna Maria to Benjamin at Shifnal School, 22 Apr 1828, in which she asks Benjamin to give 'best love' to his brother William. He was then twenty-four, so may have been an usher there, though this is speculation.

132 SA, 1987/56/28. Letter, Benjamin Wright, junior, to Edward. 28 Feb 1829.

sympathise with my dear Sister & the whole of you, in so unexpected and disturbing an event. The loss of a Son and Brother of such rare and amiable endowments would at any time cause you the deepest affliction, but at the moment when that of his beloved Father is still fresh in your minds is indeed doubly heavy, and must be a shock of such a nature as scarcely to admit of consolation, unless a firm assurance of his being removed to another & happier World will afford it. 'Twas the will of Heaven he should not be corrupted by the Vices or harassed by the cares of this World and in its Wisdom and Goodness removed him to a better.

Be pleased to remember me most affectionately to your Mother and Sisters, and believe me Dear Edward, Most sincerely yours,

Ben[j] Wright

Edinburgh, Feb 28th 1829.

People of the Nineteenth Century were no strangers to death. In 1841 the expectation of life at birth was only just over forty years and most people would be dead before they reached sixty-five.[133] But the deaths of William at fifty-six and his son at twenty-four, added to the loss of Mary as a baby and Richard in his teens, all within the space of fourteen years, would have strained the feelings of the strongest of late Georgian families.

Hard though it was for the Edwards family to bear these sorrows, the world was relentlessly changing as commerce, industry and democracy progressed, and the medical profession was changing with it. Doctors educated in the new sciences rather than the classics were rejecting the teaching of the ancients and, as the Enlightenment, in its search for truth, widened mankind's knowledge of the natural world, the

---

133   Charlton, J. and Murphy, M., *The Health of Adult Britain, 1841-1994*, p18.

profession shed the shackles of traditional thought. It became clear that Edward had been right to take the LSA, because by doing so he cast off the ancient customs of his apothecary forebears in favour of the science-based skills of medicine, surgery and midwifery. However saddened he may have been by the deaths of his father and brother, he could take pride in being qualified by public examination to be physician and surgeon. As the old system of apothecary-surgeons died with Benjamin and William, a new kind of medical profession was arising whose confidence grew as clinical knowledge and skills improved. Though the power to heal was still limited, this was the dawn of the medical profession that we have today. Edward mourned for his family but the future of his profession was bright.

Chapter 7

Edward in the Practice

Although the national economy recovered as new industries developed in the 1820s, iron producers in Shropshire began to face competition from larger enterprises elsewhere. In 1818 some of the Coalbrookdale furnaces were shut down and by 1820 closure of the whole works was being considered until, in the next few years, the company's fortunes were revived by making innovative artistic products. Though it has been said that the foundry had become the biggest in the world by 1852,[134] when William died in 1829 the Dale had lost its former prosperity and Edward was in sole charge of the medical business in difficult times. As economic recovery gradually took hold, however, he was able to employ an assistant and, as the roads improved, he bought a gig[135] which made travelling easier when he visited his patients. What had previously been his 'business' could now more properly be called his 'practice' because of his new status as 'physician and surgeon'.

Edward had hardly become accustomed to his new status when, in 1829, he was embroiled in a most extraordinary medico-legal case that must surely have tested both his skills and his conscience.[136] The Cureton family, who were his patients, lived in Teakettle Row, one of the terraces built by the Coalbrookdale Company for its workers and

---

134 Victoria County History of Shropshire, pp 50-51.

135 A light two-wheeled one-horse Carriage (OED). Such as vehicle would have cost about £12 in Edward's time, and would have been subject to a tax of £3.17s a year. Road tax is not new!

136 Gatrell, V.A.C., *The Hanging Tree: execution and the English people 1770-1868*, Oxford University Press, 1994, pp 447-493. I am much indebted to the author for his account and legal analysis of this case.

situated only a few yards from Edward's home and surgery. Richard Cureton was a puddler[137] who, with his wife Sarah, had three daughters: Mary, Ann and Elizabeth. By 1829, the older sisters had married and moved away, leaving twenty-four-year-old Elizabeth at home. Sixty or seventy people lived in the six cottages of Teakettle Row, whose thin walls allowed the neighbours to overhear the various noises of family life. Lacking space indoors, the children played where they could, including the scrap of land in front of Rose Hill. Though Edward may not have been on personal terms with the Cureton family, he would have known them as patients and seen Elizabeth growing up.

Elizabeth Cureton had made friends with several men in varying degrees of intimacy, among whom was John Noden, an odd-job man who lodged nearby and occasionally worked for Edward's uncle, Peter Wright. One night in June 1829, Noden called on Elizabeth but was rebuffed and a noisy fracas ensued in which a window was broken. Undeterred, three days later Noden again appeared at the Cureton's house, this time at nine o'clock in the evening. Though the family had gone to bed Elizabeth went downstairs, let Noden in and, as both later admitted, engaged in sexual intimacy on the parlour floor. Premarital sexual relationships were commonplace in the Dale where evening calls for this purpose were euphemistically termed 'night-visiting'. Many such liaisons must have occurred without the drastic consequences that ensued in this case.

No one witnessed this intimacy between Noden and Elizabeth, though if any voices had been raised her parents who were upstairs in a tiny house would surely have heard them. The next day Elizabeth confessed to her mother that she had been with Noden and then took to her bed. That evening Edward was called in to see her and was told that she had been visited by Noden and that there had been sexual intimacy. He found her to be 'feverish' and noticed bruises on her body

---

137 Puddlers operated the puddling furnaces in the process of making wrought iron, Michael Darby, personal communication.

but was not allowed to examine her genitals because, it was said, 'there had been no penetration'. The following day he was called again because the parish constable, Walters, had advised the Curetons to view the incident as rape. Edward's medical education had included forensic science so he knew what signs to look for. This time he was allowed to do the necessary examination but, because forty-eight hours had passed since the alleged event, he could find no convincing evidence of rape. Meanwhile the Curetons had been in touch with Noden, using the constable's advice about rape to persuade him to negotiate a settlement which might involve marriage, money or Noden paying Edward's bill rather than face a criminal charge. It is also possible that Constable Walters framed his advice in the hope that legal action would ensue for which he would be paid. Noden realised he was under pressure to 'do the honourable thing' but did not believe he would be charged with rape.

When Elizabeth felt able to leave her bed ten days later, she and her mother walked several miles to Benthall village to lay a charge against Noden before the magistrate, who referred it to the petty sessions at Much Wenlock. The Wenlock magistrates took evidence from Edward and seem to have been convinced by his scepticism about the claim. Nevertheless they bound Noden over to answer for attempted rape at the next quarter sessions, where the magistrates considered the case too serious for them and referred it to the Shrewsbury Assize. The charge then became actual, not merely attempted, rape. The difference was crucial because attempted rape was only a minor offence whereas rape was punishable by hanging. The awful truth dawned upon the hapless Noden that though he and Elizabeth had only done what comes naturally, a charge of rape meant that he would face trial for his life. It was little comfort to know that only one in five men accused of rape were convicted, that their sentences were often commuted or that there had been no execution for rape in Shrewsbury in the last thirty years.

At the Assizes the judge, Sir John Vaughan, and eighteen notable gentlemen of the county assembled as a Grand Jury, heard the King's Proclamation and paraded in their finery through the streets of Shrewsbury. It was an opportunity for a crowd of its sensation-seeking inhabitants to see justice being dispensed. On the first two days of the Assize the judge heard twenty-nine cases, mostly of petty larceny but also horse-stealing (sentence of death), house breaking (seven years' transportation) and manslaughter (fine of a shilling in mitigating circumstances). Of the twelve cases heard on the first day, five of the eight men found guilty were sentenced to death. When Noden's trial began, the courtroom was full of excited people who had discovered that the charge was to be actual rape. Because of the sexual nature of the charge, women were ordered to leave the court so Elizabeth was the only woman in a room full of men, including the colourfully robed and bewigged judge and four black-gowned attorneys, two for the prosecution and two for the defence. Unlike the cases so briefly tried on the previous day, the spectators of Noden's trial would see justice being weighed in the balance for a full nine hours.

Counsel for the prosecution said that, unlike previous friendly dalliances with Elizabeth, on this occasion Noden forced himself on an unwilling and defenceless woman. It was alleged that in her distress she screamed so loudly that she woke her mother who came downstairs to find the offence being committed — though the neighbours heard nothing. For the defence Edward testified that when first called to see her he was not allowed to carry out a genital examination because Elizabeth had told him that Noden 'had not effected his purpose'. The defence also alleged that Elizabeth was so disreputable that she could never refuse sexual advances and that there had been attempts to negotiate a financial compromise. Testimony to Noden's good character was given by several witnesses, including Peter Wright, four farmers and an innkeeper. In summing up, the judge conceded that there were 'some inconsistencies in the prosecution's case', but that 'all the evidence tending to the prisoner's conviction remained unshaken'. Having been given this broad hint that they should find the accused guilty, the jury (farmers, shopkeepers, tailors and a shoemaker) came to their decision within thirty minutes — 'Guilty, with a recommendation to mercy'. The judge ignored the recommendation and sentenced Noden to hang.

In his evidence Edward described his examination of Elizabeth and attempted to report a conversation with the constable which might have helped Noden, but was cut short by both prosecution and defence attorneys. His evidence was therefore less convincing than he intended. The judge noticed Edward's frustration at the attorneys' behaviour and, as an educated witness, invited him to a private conference after the case was concluded. The judge then ordered the execution to be delayed, perhaps intending to give time for Edward to raise an appeal, which he did. Within a few days eight men had agreed to swear affidavits before magistrates about their own sexual adventures with Elizabeth. Edward, who knew she had previously suffered from a venereal disease, also swore an affidavit, as did one of the jurors at the trial and three of the Curetons' neighbours. A petition was signed by 192 respectable people of Madeley, including some of the Darby family, Peter Wright, five local doctors and several gentlemen, all testifying to Noden's good character and their belief in his innocence. The petition was presented to Judge Vaughan, who referred it to the Home Secretary, Robert Peel. Noden's sentence was commuted to transportation to New South Wales or Van Diemen's Land (Tasmania), as were those of all the others condemned at the Assize and within days they were all in the hulk *Dolphin* at Chatham awaiting transportation. Thus was the jury's 'recommendation to mercy' conceded.

Noden's supporters in Coalbrookdale believed he was innocent and launched a second appeal. This time it was addressed to the King and signed by 398 people, including magistrates, town clerks, the Darbys, farmers, physicians and accountants. Despite the support of so many respectable citizens, this was only one of the two thousand appeals that reached the Home Office every year and it failed to persuade Peel of Noden's innocence. However, Peel did accept that Noden had been encouraged in his advances and therefore ordered that he should remain in one of the hulks at Chatham rather than be transported. Despite this pointless concession Noden was sent to Bermuda with nine hundred other convicts. Many of them perished from the hard labour, dysentery or yellow fever in Bermuda's filthy prisons but somehow Noden survived for twenty years. In 1850 he was granted a 'ticket-of leave', or parole, and returned to Coalbrookdale, where he died in 1873.

What can we make of Edward's part in this story? It must have taken much of his time, both examining Elizabeth and giving evidence to the Wenlock magistrates and the Assize. Edward probably knew Noden as a patient and also as the odd-job man who had worked for Peter Wright and maybe for the Edwards family. Edward had a degree of loyalty to both parties and if he favoured one it might adversely affect the other. Furthermore, if he gave a frank account of Elizabeth's medical history, it might be seen as a breach of confidentiality. According to Percival's 1803 book on Medical Ethics,[138] he would have been obliged to give evidence with 'discretion ... with the most scrupulous regard to fidelity and honour', but this was years before doctors were accountable to a disciplinary body that could reprimand them for unethical behaviour. In Edward's conversation with Sir John Vaughan after the trial, the judge may well have delayed the execution to allow time for Edward to organise an appeal: would this be collusion? Edward may have disapproved of the conduct of the trial and the casual way in which Noden was sentenced to death and, as a prominent member of the local community, he would have been well-placed to collect the necessary signatures. Allowing for changing attitudes over time, the reader may wish to contrast the increasingly logical methods being adopted in medicine with the peremptory actions of the law and the blatant disregard of Robert Peel's order forbidding transportation.

---

138 Percival, Thomas, *Medical Ethics,* London, 1803, p 30.

Little more than a year after the Noden case, Britain was engulfed by a dangerous epidemic — Asiatic cholera. The disease had long been known in India but with increasing travel it had spread westwards to Europe. In Britain it first appeared at Sunderland in 1831 and reached London in 1832 where seven thousand of its million inhabitants died. One of the ways it spread was by traffic on canals and rivers and, by that route, in April 1832, it reached Broseley, on the opposite side of the River Severn to Coalbrookdale, and by August it had moved upstream to Shrewsbury. Sufferers would feel cold and ill, suffer profuse diarrhoea, their limbs would become blue and their faces develop a congested appearance suggesting 'choler', a diagnostic term still in common use at that time, hence the name. A person could be well one day and dead from dehydration and exhaustion the next. The sudden onset and rapid deaths caused great alarm. In Bilston, twenty miles from Coalbrookdale, it was said that 'the appalling visitation has raged to a most frightful extent in defiance of all means to stop its progress, and is now paying no deference to persons or circumstances'.[139] Numerous useless schemes to prevent or cure it were proposed, including an imaginative but ineffective range of quack medicines and an army order for soldiers to wear scarlet flannel next to the skin. Unfortunately the medical profession's treatment with purges and emetics was no more successful.

It was clear that nation-wide action was necessary if the epidemic was to be halted but, at this time, there was no department of health and no organisation to meet such an emergency.[140] Late in 1831 the Privy Council convened a Board of Health in London, consisting of physicians and laymen, which ordered that '... in every town and village there should be a local board of health'. Such boards would consist of magistrates, clergymen, several of the principal inhabitants

---

139 *Salopian Journal,* 'Cholera', 29 Aug 1832.

140 Smith, L., Shropshire in the First Cholera Epidemic, *Transaction of the Shropshire Archaeological and History Society,* Vol LXXXIV, 2009, pp. 72-82.

and two or more medical practitioners who would correspond with the London Board of Health.

A local board was set up in Shrewsbury by the Borough Corporation in 1831 at the instigation of the mayor — not by the parish councils under the Poor Law as intended by the Privy Council. Unfortunately, personal antagonism between the town clerk and one of the infirmary physicians, Dr J. Proud Johnson, resulted in acrimonious and ineffective meetings. There was disagreement as to whether there should be physicians on the board and, if so, what their duties would be and whether they should be paid. The Corporation saw the board's duties as publicising advice, collecting statistics and organising local dispensaries for the treatment of the poor. Those who could afford to be treated by their usual medical practitioners would not be the concern of the board. Notices about prevention and suitable diets appeared, such as this:

> Choose dry food; avoid slops; be sparing in eating fruit especially if unripe; avoid pickled fish, lobsters and crabs; and remember that 'Pop, Lemonade, and Cider and all that sort of trash' are very unsafe.'[141]

People were told to report any 'indisposition of stomach or bowels' to a doctor as soon as possible and to avoid all medicines advertised as preventives as *there is no preventive* [original italics]. This well-intentioned advice was little use so long as the cause of the disease and its means of spread remained unknown and was no more than a shot in the dark. In fact, proper prevention lies in good hygiene and effective sanitation which were sadly lacking at this time, but at least it was an opportunity for the medical profession to denigrate the quacks.

Lacking confidence in the mayor's board, Shrewsbury physicians called a meeting of the 'Faculty', ie all qualified medical practitioners, and Edward Edwards was one of twenty-two men from all over the

---

141 SA, Watton's Cuttings, Vol 2, p. 398.

county who attended.[142] Meanwhile, anxiety was rising in Dawley and its neighbouring community of Coalbrookdale because many of their inhabitants were in contact with people in the Black Country where the epidemic was raging. After 'due notice' had been given in Dawley parish church, a meeting was convened that set up a local board. Much of Edward's practice lay in Dawley parish so, as parish boundaries were no barrier to disease, he was enlisted as one of the four medical members of the Dawley Board along with two clergymen, six gentlemen and the ironmasters Abraham and Alfred Darby and William Botfield.

In September, Dawley Parish Council resolved that:

> £50 be granted to the treasurer of the board of health
> to be placed at their disposal for defraying any expenses
> which may be incurred by the said board of health.

The board was to be accountable to the parish council for this money and any unspent cash was to be returned. A hospital for cholera victims was set up in unused industrial buildings,[143] but there is no further mention of cholera in the Dawley minutes. Some idea of the activity of the boards may be gathered from the example of the Broseley board whose records partially survive.[144] The parish was divided into three areas, each of which had a surgeon, but later the areas were combined under a single surgeon.[145] Inspectors were appointed to identify houses that were dilapidated and 'in a disgusting state of filth' and likely to harbour the disease. They were to be cleansed and whitewashed internally and heaps of dung and sewage, euphemistically

---

142 Smith, L., Shropshire in the First Cholera Epidemic, p 75.

143 Smith, L., Shropshire in the First Cholera Epidemic, p 78.

144 SA, 7/77, Meeting of Broseley Board of Health.

145 SA, 7537/2/7, Letter from William Fifield.

called 'nuisances', were to be removed. The board bought seven cholera lamps for fumigation of houses at a cost of £1.1.0, though they were probably useless. They also had to compensate sufferers for the destruction of their property: John Unitt's property was worth £7 2s 3d, including two feather beds (£4), a straw mattress (7s 6d), a pair of stays, stockings and some 'old clothes' among other goods. His representatives were compensated with money for one new bed, worth £2, not two, because as he had died he would not need one.[146]

Deaths of people who did not belong in the parish caused difficulties, because they were not eligible for relief. Peter Wright was involved in one case of this kind.[147] James Wood of Chetwynd died of cholera, leaving a wife, Elizabeth, and four children, all under twelve years old. Though James Wood had 'been relieved of thirty shillings' by Chetwynd parish where he had previously lived, the widow and children were now chargeable to Madeley, which Peter Wright had to confirm before a magistrate.

Fortunately, the epidemic was not as severe in Shropshire as elsewhere. For example, one doctor reported thirty-three cases in three months of whom only four died.[148] This relatively low death rate may have been because the houses were less overcrowded and insanitary than in other places though there was plenty of room for improvement; or it may have been due to intervention by the Established Church which reminded the devout that 'to-morrow it may be too late to repent' and published prayers to be used 'during the Continuance of that grievous disease with which several Places in this Kingdom are at this Time visited'.[149] Whether from human action, divine power or the natural course of all epidemics, by the end of 1832 this one had faded away.

---

146 SA, 151/3937/3, Account of John Unitt.

147 SA, WB/H/1/1/1/127, Settlement examination by Peter Wright.

148 SA, 7537/2/8, un-named medical officer's account.

149 SA, Watton's Cuttings, Vol 2, p. 397.

One of the first to comment on the unjust effect of the epidemic was the radical reformer and pamphleteer William Cobbett (1763-1835). In a piece reprinted in the *Shrewsbury Chronicle* in March 1832, he reiterated the widely accepted view that diseases 'generally proceed from poverty and filth'. The cholera epidemic was just the same as many in the past, he said, and such disasters always affected the poor more than the rich.[150] He was sure that 'the people are poorer and more filthy than they ever were before' and laid the blame on the government and the 'confusion in which the affairs of this great country now are'. He acknowledged that the rich were raising money to 'provide the means of giving proper food, raiment, bedding, medicines and fuel to the poor ... and to cleanse the habitations of those who are unable to do it themselves'. But, he asked, why had this not been done before? Because, he believed, the intensity of the epidemic had forced the rich to see that they, too, were at risk from the squalor in which they allowed the poor to exist.

The local boards may have been effective in slowing, if not halting, the spread of the disease but they had a more durable consequence. By drawing attention to the appalling sanitary arrangements in the rapidly growing towns where many shoddy new houses were being built, the epidemic forced people to confront the matter of sanitation. The boards brought men (no women yet) together to seek solutions to a problem shared by rich and poor alike and were thus the first step in a process that eventually led to legislation on standards of building and sanitation. Cobbett's comments on the 'filth diseases' were prescient of Chadwick's Report on the Sanitary Condition of the Labouring Population[151] which exposed the squalid conditions of the poor and led to the Public Health campaigns of the 1840s and 1850s. Public alarm during the cholera epidemic of 1831-2 was renewed when it

---

150 *Shrewsbury Chronicle*, 2 Mar 1832.

151 Chadwick, E., *Report on the Sanitary Condition of the Labouring Population of Great Britain,* Presented to the House of Lords, 1842.

burst out again in 1849 and Dr John Snow famously demonstrated that the disease was spread through the water supply. Parliament was forced to ensure that clean water and effective sewers were provided. Good *can* come from evil — sometimes.

If 1832 was significant in sanitary reform, it was momentous in politics because of the so-called Great Reform Act. Widening the electorate of the House of Commons had been discussed intermittently since the end of the Civil War in 1649, but little had changed. A note in the *Salopian Journal* in 1831 reported that between 1782 and 1830 the House of Commons had debated the matter 25 times but the motions had always been defeated or withdrawn.[152] The concept of democracy based on a wide franchise had been viewed with deep suspicion in Britain during the French Revolution but, by the 1820s, pressure of public opinion resulted in action. Until then the Commons had been elected by a mere 400,000 property owners, and the buying of votes and other corrupt practices were commonplace. After heated disagreements and debates *An Act to amend the representation of the people in England and Wales* received Royal Assent on 7 June 1832 which, although only concerned with parliamentary elections, also had effects in many areas of society including medical profession. The Act only increased the electorate from 400,000 to 650,000 'male persons', about five per cent of the adult population, but it challenged the assumption that an unrepresentative and elite minority could determine the fortunes of the much larger majority. Two years later representative democracy was introduced into local government by the Municipal Boroughs Act, and before long organisations such as the Chartist Movement were arguing for the franchise to be extended to non-property owners. Majority decision-making became commonplace, and was soon adopted in the medical profession, as we shall see later.

The cholera epidemic prompted another parliamentary reform by concentrating attention on support of the poor and sick, not

---

152   *Salopian Journal,* 23 Feb 1831.

particularly for their own sake but because, as Cobbett had realised, they were an economic liability and harboured the 'fever nests' from which infectious diseases could spread throughout the population. Under the antiquated Tudor system of poor relief, parishes were responsible for relieving their own poor by doles of money or admission to a 'poor house'. The 1834 Poor Law Amendment Act amalgamated individual parishes into 'Unions', thereby spreading the burden over larger populations and improving administrative efficiency. They were run by Boards of Guardians responsible to the central Poor Law Commission in London. Guardians set a levy on properties to support the sick and disabled in their homes and to provide workhouses for the destitute. This latter turned out to be an oppressive and inhumane regime, as Charles Dickens famously described in *Oliver Twist*, yet some of its provisions are relevant to the development of medical care and the story of the Coalbrookdale doctors.

Every Union had one or more part-time medical officers whose remuneration covered their salaries, out of which they had to supply and pay for all the medicines, splints and dressings they used (though, curiously, not hernia trusses). Unsurprisingly, the medicines provided were usually the cheapest available. The so-called 'New Poor Law' was intended to be a nationwide system for the sick poor to be treated by qualified doctors at public expense and is therefore a distant forerunner of the National Health Service, where treatment is 'free at the point of need'. Benjamin Wright had been an Overseer of the Poor, and in their time William and Edward were both medical officers to Madeley parish under the old system. The new arrangements did not reach Shropshire until 1836 when the commissioner for Shropshire, William Day, grouped its three hundred parishes into eleven Unions. One of these, the Madeley Union, was formed by amalgamating the parish of Madeley with several of its neighbours. While waiting for Day's decision all nine local doctors in the area of the new union would have been anxious about how it would affect them: some would gain

EDWARD IN THE PRACTICE

if they were appointed to be Union medical officers but others would lose their previous incomes from parish work. Edward wrote to his brother Benjamin:

> I expect an alteration in the parishes, the Poor Law Commission is in this neighbourhood & has thrown into an Union M[uch] Wenlock, Broseley, Madeley and Dawley with several of less importance, how it will affect me I do not know. Madeley poor House will be the principle receptacle.[153]

Later he reported:

> Mr Procter [of Ironbridge] has been appointed to the parishes of Madeley district, to the great mortification of his competitors. Thursfield has engaged both Broseley and Wenlock districts, Brookes and Bowyer had bargained together & consequently were disappointed.[154]

Whether Edward was one of Procter's competitors for the appointment is not known: if he was he must have been as disappointed as his colleagues Brookes and Bowyer because such an appointment could provide a small but steady income to supplement their other earnings.

The rising demand for representation in government was mirrored in the medical profession. By the 1830s there were about twenty thousand trained doctors in England and Wales, most of whom had taken the LSA examination or were exempt from it because they were already in practice and, like Edward, had styled themselves 'Physician and

---

153 SA, 1987/56/7, Letter, Edward to Benjamin.

154 SA, 1987/56/11, Letter, Edward to Benjamin.

Surgeon'. But there was still no central organisation to represent their views or argue their case for reform. The regular medical profession became seriously overcrowded and there were thousands of more-or-less educated irregulars of varying ability. Competition for custom was severe but, although doctors clamoured for protection from the rivalry of allegedly incompetent competitors, they had no means of representing their demands to parliament. The only organisations that could do so were the three London corporations: the Royal College of Physicians, the Royal College of Surgeons and the Society of Apothecaries, none of which were concerned with the thousands of new general practitioners. As in national and local government, a direct and democratic system of representation was necessary.

At this time many small locally-based groups were formed to discuss matters of scientific interest and one of them, the Yorkshire Philosophical Society, realised the advantages to be gained by communicating with each other. In 1831 that Society proposed that similar organisations should be 'linked ... in unity of purpose, common participation and division of labour'.[155] This led to the foundation of the British Association for the Advancement of Science, whose second meeting, in Oxford in 1832, was attended by the thirty-eight-year-old Worcester physician, Dr (later Sir) Charles Hastings. His experience there encouraged an idea that had already been taking shape in his mind: that an association should be formed to represent provincial doctors and counter-balance the powerful London medical bodies. Hastings proposed that a new society be founded that would be open to *all* medical men. On 1st May 1832 a prospectus was published in the *Midland Reporter,* a journal popular with doctors, that acknowledged that although much progress had been made in discovering 'the laws of nature' it was difficult to disseminate such knowledge amongst so many practitioners. Accordingly it was proposed to:

---

155   McMenemey, W. H., *The Life and Times of Sir Charles Hastings,* Edinburgh and London, E & S Livingstone, 1959, p. 74.

Associate the Provincial Medical Practitioners of England, or at least as many as can be brought to rally around a common centre, in a comprehensive Institution.[156]

Progress was fast. Within eleven weeks, on 19th July, fifty doctors from the Midlands — Worcester, Cheltenham, Oxford and Bristol and elsewhere — met at the Worcester Infirmary. They resolved to found the Provincial Medical and Surgical Association (PMSA) which was to be open to every qualified medical and surgical practitioner in Britain and to be run on democratic lines, and in which all members would have the right to vote. National meetings were to be held annually and branches were to be formed throughout the country to give ordinary practitioners a democratic voice in the development of their own profession. A Shropshire branch of the PMSA was formed at Shrewsbury in 1838 and Edward was soon to become a member. One frequently debated issue was the failure of the Apothecaries Act to defend qualified doctors from unqualified competitors. Another was the miserly remuneration and oppressive terms of service of Union medical officers. As the PMSA gathered strength it formulated powerful arguments for better regulation of medical services and began to present its case to Parliament.

The creation of a national network of PMSA branches was a considerable achievement at a time when communication was unreliable and travel slow and complicated. It would be difficult for a doctor in Kent or Lincolnshire to attend a meeting in Worcester, even if he had heard about it. Although the radical medical journal, *The Lancet,* had been founded in 1823, its reach was limited. National events were difficult to advertise effectively because newspapers were mostly local and there was no cheap and dependable postal system until, in 1840, Rowland Hill introduced the penny post. At the

---

156 McMenemey, W. H., *The Life and Times of Sir Charles Hastings,* p 89.

same time, the railway network expanded rapidly and attendance at meetings became more practicable, whether local, regional or national. Edward could ride in his gig to a local railway station, catch a train to Shrewsbury, attend a PMSA meeting followed by a formal dinner and return the same evening.

Not only did the PMSA exchange and publish scientific information, but it gathered the medico-political concerns of the profession and represented them to government, especially in the areas of professional education and protection from unqualified competitors. In 1855 it changed its name to The British Medical Association, which is now the professional association which represents the great majority of doctors in Britain.[157] The newly-named BMA continued the campaign and, after nineteen fruitless attempts to introduce a parliamentary bill, it achieved its purpose in 1858 with the passing of the Medical Act. This created the General Medical Council (GMC) and required all qualified medical men to enter their names on the new Medical Register held by the GMC, which would oversee the regulation of professional conduct. The Register, which was little more than a list of doctors who had passed the test of competence, did nothing to diminish the activities of untrained rivals and it earned the *soubriquet* 'The Quacks' Charter'. However, the Medical Act, brought about by democratic processes within the profession and parliament, did at last establish the profession as a legal entity and introduced the regulatory system of the medical profession today.

The scientific and industrial revolutions that erupted between 1770 and 1830 encouraged a more rational approach to medical diagnosis and treatment, and the prosperous new middle classes began to buy the services of an increasingly confident profession. Modern scientific

---

157 McMenemey, W. H., *The Life and Times of Sir Charles Hastings,* p 407. For many years the title 'British Medical Association' had been used by a small group in London which had been dissolved by the early 1850s, and so became available for use by the Provincial Medical and Surgical Association.

medicine could not have developed without the discoveries of men such as Priestley, Davy and Faraday, and the prosperity generated by such brilliant entrepreneurs or inventors as the Darbys, Trevithick, Boulton and Watt. Nor could Britain's fortunes have flourished without the arduous, injurious and lowly paid labour of untold thousands of men, women and children in mines and mills and manufactories.

The 1820s and 1830s were decades of great change. For Edward, the Coalbrookdale doctor of the time, the Cureton case focussed attention on professional values and his belief in justice; for the profession its greater knowledge and cohesion called for a system of medical ethics. Cholera brought Edward and his colleagues together in the face of a danger to the public health and demonstrated the urgent need for sanitary reform. And the growth of democracy, communication and travel enabled the medical profession to unite in common cause to achieve its establishment as a legal entity. Doctors were still far from effective in the prevention or cure of disease but progress was being made, albeit slowly, in professional cooperation and scientific knowledge. By 1858, medicine was beginning to be the coherent and rational exercise we expect it to be today.

But at home the Edwards family had other concerns. Anna Maria and Fanny were now young ladies — and the teenage Benjamin was about to go to London to study medicine.

Chapter 8

Benjamin in London

After the deaths in the 1820s of William senior, Richard and William junior, the Edwards family must have hoped for better times. In 1831 Elizabeth settled to her widow's role, Fanny, now twenty-three, recovered from the typhus that had laid her low three years earlier, and twenty-one-year-old Anna Maria completed her education. The teenage Benjamin would soon finish school and go to London to study. But their hopes of better times were shattered.

Fanny, full of expectation, took a post at New Park House School in Cheltenham under the proprietor Miss Ferriday.[158] She said the school was a 'paradise' and the other ladies there, Miss Henderson and Miss Finch, were 'amiable, affectionate and kind', but within weeks she was hurrying home following some disturbance. Evidently Miss Finch wrote to Elizabeth about it, but her letter has not survived so we can only guess what the problem was. The family were worried by what they heard. Anna Maria wrote to Fanny immediately saying she must come home at once, regretting that she 'should have been made so uncomfortable and disappointed'. All was well for a few years then tragedy struck again. Anna Maria became ill and, in 1835, she died. Elizabeth now mourned the loss of a husband, two daughters and two sons. Sorrow laid a heavy hand on Rose Hill.

However sad the family might be, nineteen-year-old Benjamin had to look to the future and join his brother as bread-winner. He had been indentured for a five-year apprenticeship to his brother Edward in 1830 at the age of fourteen and, when that was completed in October 1835, he was ready to become a medical student in London — three years older than his brother Edward had been when he had started.

---

158   SA, 1987/56/31, Letter, Fanny to Anna Maria.

Because the medical world was developing rapidly, his studies would be far more extensive than Edward's, let alone his father William's forty years earlier. Diagnosis now required detailed physical examination of the patient for signs of disease as old assumptions were abandoned, and students had to study the rapidly expanding science of chemistry rather than botany. In the course of time medical education became a major faculty in the University of London as the hospital schools integrated with that newly-founded institution.

Benjamin set off for London in 1835 just as these changes were happening. The London to Birmingham railway was still unfinished so he boarded the horse-drawn coach *Nimrod* at Shifnal.[159] He travelled outside in 'pleasant weather with occasional rain', 'got a good dinner' at Dunstable and arrived at Holborn at 10 o'clock the same evening. A man from Corbyn's, the pharmaceutical wholesaler Edward dealt with, was there to meet him and carry his luggage to lodgings arranged with Mr and Mrs Mayfield at 300 Holborn. Next day, he did some business for his brother about supplies of drugs and honey (a common ingredient of medicines) and started looking for permanent lodgings. Everything and everybody seemed very strange because of 'the sudden change from such a place as Coalbrookdale to noisy Holborn' and he always had to be on his guard against pick-pockets. He found two comfortable rooms at the house of Mr Lipscombe, a water-filter maker, in Lamb's Conduit Street conveniently close to King's College. The rent was twelve shillings a week, to include breakfast and 'tea at whatever hour I choose', but he had to find his dinner elsewhere, usually for about ten pence. He left those lodgings after a few weeks, however, and for a while shared rooms with another student, but he found this disturbing and eventually secured a much more suitable place on his own where he would not be 'interrupted by strangers'.

Benjamin had to enrol on the necessary courses, discover where the best lectures were given and by whom and, of course, pay for them.

---

159   SA, 1987/56/23, Letter, Benjamin to Edward.

Edward made funds available for him at a bank, from which he paid £29 8s 0d to enrol at the new King's College. He later discovered that he could get a refund of £4 12s 0d when he found a 'proprietor' of the college to nominate him. He also had to join dissection classes and buy books and instruments, all of which must have been stressful for a young man unaccustomed to metropolitan life. Because postage was still costly he kept in touch with his family by sending letters with the orders and goods travelling between Coalbrookdale and Corbyn's. Sometimes letters from home were accompanied by pies and filberts, but no wine was sent to drink with them for fear of breaking the bottle.

At first Benjamin was alarmed by the commotion and dangers of the capital's streets and found it hard to organise himself. Life in the crowded metropolis was very different from his earlier experiences in the sooty seclusion of Coalbrookdale. He was not alone in struggling with the challenges of further education; a year earlier *The Lancet* had commented on the problems that might confront the newcomer:

> The medical student on arriving in London to commence his metropolitan studies will, unless guided by a friendly and experienced monitor, speedily find himself bewildered by the multiplicity of the schools and the extent of the ground over which they are spread. No less than fifty prospectuses and advertisements await his perusal.[160]

Benjamin's relationship with his brother was unusual. He was only twelve years old when their father died, so the twenty-nine-year-old Edward assumed paternal responsibility for him which they both took seriously. Edward was keen that Benjamin should lead a well-ordered life and be committed to his studies. For example, when he heard that Benjamin was sharing rooms he advised him 'not to waste time in

---

160 *The Lancet*, 1833-4, p. 3.

gossiping', and 'on no account ... let your early hours be broken [and] always be beforehand not to lend money on any excuse'.[161] He advised against burning the midnight oil: 'I do not approve of sitting up later than half past ten and always have breakfast some time earlier than is required for the lectures, for ... then you will not be inconvenienced by the dilatoriness of the landlord's servants'. He offered advice about taking the Latin examination, pickpockets, having an old coat to wear when dissecting and a box to keep it in, and being economical with money which 'is easier spent than obtained'. He also commented on a more intimate matter:

> You must pay strict attention to y^r bowels, and if they continue so inactive you may take some Ex Colc c Ex Hyosc to which may be added some Pil Camb Co & occasionally an electuary with Conf Senna et Jalap. A little Sod Tart would now and then be useful.[162]

A better system of lavatories might also have helped.

Most importantly, he wanted Benjamin to be thoroughly committed to his studies.

> I hope earnestly that you will be ambitious of the highest honours and leave no stone unturned to obtain them. Y^r return home will then be like a fortunate Warrior covered with Laurels. Industry and perseverance will overcome any difficulty. Try to emulate the bright traits in the characters of History. Napoleon was accustomed

---

161 SA, 1957/56/4, Letter from Edward to Benjamin. 'Be beforehand' = take care.

162 a) Extracts of Colchicine (Colc) are from Autumn crocus and of Hyoscine (Hyosc) from Henbane: b) a pill containing Camboge vegetable resin: Senna and Jalap vegetable purgatives: c) sodium tartrate or Rochelle salt, an effervescent solution. Beasley, H. *The Book of Prescriptions,* London, John Churchill, 1854.

to say that nothing was done while anything remained undone. In wishing you to be ambitious of distinction amongst your Fellows I by no means wish you to obtain it by any of the low arts of sycophancy or dissimulation, but in every action of life to be guided by a broad Principle of Honor [*sic*] and Integrity ... You will learn devoted loyalty to your King & reverence for the sacred institutions of your Country.

This was good brotherly and fatherly advice to a young student living away from home for the first time and more constructive than some that Edward himself had received. The reader may recall his mother's anxiety about him falling into the frozen Thames and his father's view that theatres were 'beneath the Notice of any man of Sense and Business'. At home Benjamin's family were 'much gratified by the progress you have made since leaving home' and his mother could 'think and talk of nothing but Benjamin'. But the young man did not always rise to the challenges his brother set for his future. Having lost his father at twelve years old, he may have been confused by the influences of an anxious mother, three older sisters, a strict and vigilant brother and the regime of a Nineteenth-Century boarding school.[163] His teenage years had been difficult and he had an adolescent tendency to rebel that contrasted with his willingness to turn to Edward for help.

Edward had two periods of study in London, once before and again after the Apothecaries Act of 1815. His first visit lasted only a few months during which he attended lectures and 'walked the wards' but took no examination. After the Apothecaries Act he had returned to study for the LSA examination despite his father's doubts about its significance. Students had to arrange their own attendance at the various dispensaries, hospitals and private schools that were

---

163 Benjamin was at school in the 1830s. Charles Dickens published *Nicholas Nickleby*, which describes the appalling conditions of Dotheboys Hall, in 1838.

accredited for the LSA and, by the time Benjamin arrived, lectures at the recently-founded University and King's Colleges were also available. The medical schools at hospitals such as St Thomas's and The London did not set examinations themselves and rules for medical degrees in the new university were still being developed. Benjamin therefore had to plan where to study for a curriculum that was greatly expanded both in time and subject matter compared to that which Edward had experienced. Table 8.1. (overleaf) shows the differences.

The new requirements included an additional forty-five lectures in each of Chemistry, *Materia Medica,* and Botany, and an extra year of clinical experience in both hospital and dispensary which had previously been alternatives.[164] Studies in physiology, anatomy and dissection had to conform to the regulations of the Royal College of Surgeons. It was a much longer and more intensive course than Edward had undergone, although during the long vacation from July to October Benjamin could return to the relative peace of Coalbrookdale and help in the practice.

Inevitably the longer course was more expensive; consequently Edward wanted to ensure that Benjamin was committed to his studies and subsequent work in the practice — if that was what he eventually decided on:

> You appear to be placed in a very advantageous school & will only require assiduity to raise yourself in public estimation which is the road to fortune & which I sincerely wish you may attain. I recommend you not to divert your mind in any degree from the subject, you must make it a pleasure & then you will not want for recreation. A man should make his business his amusement.[165]

---

164 Steggall, J., *A manual for students preparing for examination at Apothecaries Hall or other medical examinations.*

165 SA, 1987/56/6, Letter, Edward to Benjamin, 17 Jan. 1836.

Table 8.1
Changes in requirements for entry to the LSA examination

Courses and Lectures	Edward in 1814 — Number of courses	Benjamin in 1835 — Number of courses (90 hours each)
Anatomy and Physiology	2	**2 or conform to R C Surgeons regulation**
Anatomical demonstration	0	**2 or conform to R C Surgeons regulation**
Principles and Practice of Medicine	2	2
Chemistry	1	2
Materia Medica (pharmacology)	1	2
Forensic medicine	0	**50 hours in second year**
Midwifery and Diseases of Women and Children	0	2
Botany	0	**50 lectures**
Clinical Experience		
Attendance at the practice of a public hospital, infirmary or dispensary	6 months	**Total of 18 months, 12 at hospital with 60 or more beds, plus 6 months at dispensary**
Apprenticeship to an apothecary	5 years	5 years
All candidates to be competent in Latin.		Additional requirements in **bold**.

This was good advice, no doubt, though Edward may have intended to imply that theatres were not the place for Benjamin's recreation any more than it had been for Edward years before.

Edward's letters frequently contain advice on books, on which lectures to hear and on how to get the best from them. Benjamin apparently believed that new and well-reviewed books were essential to his studies but Edward reminded him that the mere possession of a book does not instil knowledge: it must be read. In his view such purchases were 'a waste of money ... you will hear much puffing of Books by different parties & more frequently by those who are little competent to appreciate their value'. Books should be bought direct from the publisher to obtain the best discounts. Benjamin must attend the best lecturers, too. Edward recommended hearing William Brande's lectures at Great Windmill Street because Brande's book on chemistry and *materia medica* was highly regarded. He also recommended William Lawrence, a controversial figure who had had a bitter dispute with the eminent surgeon John Abernethy to whom he had once been apprenticed. The controversy was about the nature of human life: was it an entirely spiritual phenomenon explicable by religious belief, or a purely physical one susceptible to scientific enquiry? Lawrence championed the cause of scientists who were not afraid to challenge religious and social conventions or to speak what they believed to be the truth.[166] This was to swim against the tide because many people distrusted the scientific approach, influenced as it was by the French medical schools and therefore tainted with unacceptable revolutionary ideas.[167] Medical science and practice cannot be protected from the political and religious controversies of the day.

Despite Benjamin's good start which had 'much gratified' the family, as time went by Edward began to worry about his brother's

---

166 Oxford Dictionary of National Biography, on-line edition, accessed 12 Jun 2013.

167 Lawrence, S. *Charitable Knowledge: hospital pupils and practitioners in eighteenth century London,* pp 329-33.

commitment, mistrusting his attitude to lectures and fearing that he was 'loosing time' by delaying his dissecting studies. Students had to obtain evidence that they had attended lectures approved for the LSA curriculum, but many of them managed to get the necessary certificates without actually being present. It seems Benjamin was one such. Edward agreed that certificates were necessary, but he was adamant:

> I must caution you against the practice of omitting your attendance at your own lectures to go to hear this or that other lecturer. It will lead you into instability of habits and generate a wish for change...[168]

He had to reinforce the message later:

> I wish I could push that ridiculous notion out of your head of attending lectures to obtain certificates ... you ought to attend them for the purpose of gaining information & therefore should gain it as soon as you can. The great object will be to get as much information as will be useful hereafter. I have in former letters laid down what will prove (in Y^r future Practice) the best plan to pursue.[169]

His reasons for pressing Benjamin to get on with his studies were twofold. One was the very obvious need to make the best use of his time because the cost of living in London was a drain on the family's financial resources. The other was that Edward was exceptionally busy at this time and was unwell. It was not legally necessary for Benjamin

---

168 SA, 1978/56/4, Letter, Edward to Benjamin, Nov 25 1835.

169 SA, 1987/56/5, Letter, Edward to Benjamin.

to have passed the LSA to work in the practice because being under his brother's supervision would distinguish him from an unlicensed quack. If Benjamin was not making good use of his time in London he could be better employed at home. Edward wrote:

> I trust you will now see the importance of improving time & leave nothing undone that is likely to be useful hereafter. It is an opportunity that only offers once in a lifetime.

He was a caring brother but a hard task-master.

Edward may have underestimated the changing mood in medicine and medical education at this time. As fears of war and revolution faded in the social and political fields, steps towards democracy were being taken that led to the Great Reform Act and the Municipal Corporations Act of the 1830s — punctuated by occasional outbreaks of violence as at Peterloo and the Shropshire coalfield. Similarly in medicine, students sought to influence the way they were taught and their demands were sometimes noisily expressed. Didactic teaching and examination by figures of authority gave way to reason, evidence and scientific knowledge,

The 1830s was a decade of change. Benjamin may therefore have had misgivings about his choice of career and may have been unsettled by one particularly rebellious event that occurred shortly after his arrival, when hundreds of medical students and some of their teachers gathered in a mass protest. The meeting had been provoked by the unexpected failure in the LSA of a highly regarded student, Thomas Smith, who had been examined *viva voce* by a single examiner without a witness. The rules of the examination did not allow failed candidates to try again or appeal against their examiners' decisions, so candidates' professional prospects were seriously damaged by such failure. Unfortunately, the examiner had a grudge against Smith's teacher and it was generally believed that he was determined to expose the candidate's weakness and therefore the teacher's inadequacy. Believing the examiner to have been ill-informed and biased, Smith decided to bring the matter to the attention of the public. The following letter appeared in *The Lancet*:

> To the Court of Examiners of *The Apothecaries' Hall*
>
> Gentlemen,
> Having applied to you last night for the Licence of your Company and having been examined by one of the examiners of the Court and 'rejected', I must attribute such 'rejection' to the operation of some private feeling which I have good reason for supposing existed in the mind of my examiner. In order therefore to prove to the PROFESSION generally and to the PUBLIC that such 'rejection' was not the result of incompetency on my part I demand from you a PUBLIC EXAMINATION to be conducted in the presence of a professional audience, and I now state to you I am ready to undergo such an ordeal on any day, and at any hour which you may be pleased to appoint.
>
> I am, gentlemen, your obedient servant
> THOMAS SMITH
> 1 Jewin-crescent, Friday morning, 8th Jan. 1834
> [Original upper case emphasis]

This courageous challenge brought to light a serious issue that had been festering since 1815 when the Apothecaries Society was first charged with examining medical students for competence to practise. The widely held view that it was inappropriate for a pharmaceutical trading company with no role in medical teaching to determine the competence of future medical practitioners was fomented from week to week by *The Lancet*. From its origin as a radical medical journal in

1823, one of *The Lancet's* major objectives was reform of the medical profession including the role of the Apothecaries' Society which it disparagingly referred to as 'Rhubarb Hall'.[170] In January 1836, a 'Great Meeting of the Medical Students of London' was convened at the Crown and Anchor Tavern, scene of many such medical protest meetings.[171] *The Lancet* reported that 'nearly the whole of the medical students in London were assembled', so Benjamin may well have been among them. The high-spirited meeting was frequently punctuated by shouts of '*Hear, hear and cries of laughter*', '*No, No, go on, go on*' and '*Shame, shame*', but remained orderly, with none of the raucous misbehaviour then supposedly typical of medical students.

The meeting elected a young medical teacher, William Meade, as chairman. He alleged that 'many acts of injustice have been committed by that tyrannical body, the Apothecaries' Society', one of which had been brought to public notice by Thomas Smith who had been 'interrogated in the strangest manner'. The complaints against Smith's examiner were that he was ill-informed and out of date, and that the questions were put in 'a gruff and surly voice'. However, the agenda of the meeting was broader than that: it was to expose the inadequacies of the Apothecaries' Society as the arbiter of competence for medical practice. Debates on each of the four proposals were lively and vigorous and, despite some arguments against, were all carried overwhelmingly. The actual wording of the resolutions seems somewhat verbose to the modern reader, but can be summarised thus:

> The LSA examination was not 'conducive' to the honour of the medical profession or protection of the public, and was not an adequate test of candidates' competence. A petition demanding a remedy for this

---

170 A variety of rhubarb imported from Turkey was often prescribed as a laxative at this time, hence the innuendo.

171 *The Lancet*, 1835-6 (1), p. 668-680.

evil should be sent to parliament. Such a remedy would require that examiners should be elected by all licentiates of the Society, not appointed by the London-based and unrepresentative Council.

The thin end of a democratic wedge had been hammered into the monolith of medical education.

The Great Meeting of the Medical Students not only aired the frustrations of the students themselves and some of their teachers but, importantly, it secured the support of two MPs who were staunch advocates of medical reform. One was Henry Warburton, whose efforts in parliament to protect the profession and public from incompetent quacks greatly contributed to the Medical Act of 1858, which recognised the medical profession as a legal entity. He was unable to attend the meeting himself but enthusiastically supported the students' cause. The other was Thomas Wakley, irascible editor of *The Lancet*, whose presence at the meeting was 'received with many rounds of enthusiastic cheers'.[172] He said he was gratified to find that medical students were so active in their desire to reform the antiquated systems of the profession, and their petition to parliament would advance that cause. He called for two significant reforms. The first was that all examinations should be in public, that is, in the presence of informed persons who could judge the fairness of the proceedings and put an end to prejudiced private interrogations. The second, more radical, demand was that the LSA examination should not simply be reformed; it should be *abolished* so that it 'could no longer inflict undeserved punishment on medical students'. Wakley claimed that Thomas Smith's examination was illegal because it was not held by a quorum of the Court, as the Apothecaries' Act had prescribed, but by a single examiner who asked a series of 'paltry, miserable, manoeuvring and trick questions'. Wakley

---

172   This is how the meeting was reported in *The Lancet*, so Wakely's account may not be truly objective.

supported the proposals then being made to found a new University of London and urged the students to appoint a delegation to wait upon the Chancellor of the Exchequer who was at that time framing the rules for doing so. Medical education was embarking on its own radical, rational but peaceful revolution.

After the long vacation of 1836, Benjamin returned to London for his second year as a medical student. But all was not well. The family had to wait a long time to hear of his safe return to London, which particularly worried his mother. Edward assumed that no news was good news but suspected that Benjamin was not as committed as he should have been. The brothers seem to have had a serious disagreement, perhaps to do with the practice or some wayward act by Benjamin, although it is now impossible to know exactly what happened. Edward was forthright in his letter of 18 November 1836:

> Although I have been much hurt recently by your want of government of an irritable temper, still I can make allowance for the indiscretions of youth, & I trust for your own future advantage you will study to govern with a steady resolution the temptation to a petulant and conceited behaviour. It is the *suaviter in modo* that gains the affections & the *fortiter in re*[173] the respect and esteem of your relations and society in general: humility combined with firmness will obtain for you advantages far greater than a haughty demeanour.[174]

Edward was an experienced man advising a young one setting out in the world and his advice was now decidedly fatherly. He had once been a teenager too and was aware of the follies of youth. Edward said

---

173 Suaviter *in modo* = being gentle in manner. *Fortiter in re* = being strong in action.

174 SA, 1987/56/8, Letter, Edward to Benjamin, 18 Nov 1836.

Benjamin's 'conduct had not been pleasing on many occasions' but he trusted that his brother would eventually gain a sense of responsibility:

> It is gratifying to us to think you have not been activated by a vicious disposition, but from want of consideration or charity for the opinion of others, who, you will learn as you advance in life, have different views of the circumstances as they arise ... therefore you should endeavour to act towards others as <u>you would</u> they should act towards you [original underlining].

'Do as you would be done by' was good advice then, as now.

Despite these differences Edward continued in supportive vein about many things. He urged Benjamin to get on with his work — 'you must exert yourself to the utmost to dissect this winter' — but again warned against buying unsuitable books. He should select those needed for his examination, not speculative volumes on topics like 'theories of the nervous system'. He must sign up to study at a dispensary, go to lectures on comparative anatomy (the study of species other than humans) and be sure to attend the Hunterian Oration at the Royal College of Surgeons.[175] And, especially, he must study midwifery because that was now an important and responsible part of the duties of the general practitioner.

There was a lighter side to Edward's letters, however, and it was useful to have a contact in London. Benjamin could send copies of *The Times* or *The Standard* newspapers or, better still, *St James Chronicle* which contained two days' news. He was asked to buy some gum lancets for Edward — 'good size and moderately strong' — and an instrument for dental extractions as a present to Edward's assistant,

---

175 A lecture endowed in memory of the great anatomist John Hunter by the executors of his will in 1813, 'such oration to be expressive of the merits in comparative anatomy, physiology, and surgery'. Wikipedia, accessed 12 Jun 2013.

Lomax. He was to report the price of Cod Fish and Soles, and send lobsters and oysters — 'a peck or perhaps a few more will be a proper quantity providing the price is reasonable'.[176] They were to be sent by the night coach to Birmingham and then by the Mail to Ironbridge so as to arrive without delay.

Rumours of changes in medical education had reached Edward, who wanted to hear what was going on at the new university:

> Have you learned what kind of degrees will be granted at the new University, and whether they are intended to be merely honorary, or for qualification to supersede the other qualifications at the [Apothecaries'] Hall and College [of Surgeons]?[177]

This question has echoes of Edward's own time in London when his father, William, had regarded the LSA as 'merely honorary' evidence of completed studies. Reports of the new university hinted at things to come. Though only a provincial doctor, Edward was keen to know about developments in science and the new system of medical education:

> I should like to hear if there is any thing new in the Medical or Chemical World & if the Lancet or Gazette newspapers should contain a full account of the University and its regulations ... I should like it sent down if there is opportunity.[178]

This was not as easy as it sounded because, although oysters justified

---

176 Peck: about 2 gallons. (Concise OED): a large quantity of oysters by today's standards!

177 SA, 1987/56/5, Letter, Edward to Benjamin.

178 SA, 1987/56/9, Letter, Edward to Benjamin.

the expense of rapid delivery by the Mail, there was still no inexpensive postal service for letters or newspapers that would have to come with the supplies from Corbyn's.[179] There were other practical purchases to be made too. Edward wanted his practice equipment to be up-to-date so he asked Benjamin to enquire of the hospital surgeons which were the best 'apparatus for dislocations' and to discover the price of 'a good electrical machine and Galvanic apparatus'. Benjamin was also asked to discover the 'lowest price for ready money' for Globes at Cary's, the map-maker, and enquire if the new Ordnance Survey map of Shropshire had been finished.

While Benjamin was in London, life continued for the Edwards family and their neighbours in Coalbrookdale. One big project concerned alterations to the house at Rose Hill. William had originally leased it from Sarah Darby but, after her death in 1822, ownership passed to her friend and companion Susannah Appleby. She had modernised The Chestnuts, another house close to Rose Hill that she had inherited, and now proposed to alter Rose Hill. The house had been enlarged in 1829 by the addition of a 'cottage'[180] and other alterations were now put in hand. By November 1836, the builders had modified some rooms which were now 'very commodious', and one of the rooms had been converted to a library.[181] New furniture, including a large piece for the kitchen 8 ft high and 7 ft wide, was bought for more than £300 which Edward said was 'a serious drain'. A new portico to the front of the house and a bigger stable with two stalls were nearing completion. It was all very frustrating for Edward who said he 'dreaded using the surgery' in the house in the midst of the alterations.

---

179 Sending letters with Corbyn's despatches would save the high cost of mail before the introduction of the Penny Post.

180 SA, 1987/56/26, Letter, Richard Edwards (senior) to Edward.

181 SA, 1987/56/8, Letter, Edward to Benjamin.

Edward also wrote about the practice. His young mare was lame because the blacksmith had cut a corn too deeply (as had happened to his father's horse), which was a serious problem causing Edward to walk on his visiting rounds. In January 1836, the practice was very busy with as many as 'one hundred on the slate' (the record of current patients), and Edward often visited the same patient twice in a day. There had been 'many cases of typhus in the Dale amongst children' and several of jaundice and rheumatic fever. In March, there were as many as thirty cases of typhus at the same time, with fifteen deaths from the disease. A contemporary textbook for students described the symptoms of typhus thus:

> At first langour, chilliness and depressed spirits, with sighing and oppression in the breathing, followed by pains in the head ... confusion of thought ...pulse quick and weak ... A change in the state of the patient, named the *crisis*, is often observed on the fourteenth day.[182]

Complications such as pneumonia could occur, and the death rate could be 10-20 percent.[183]

Edward would sometimes see sixty patients a day including typhus cases, and his assistants, Lomax and Fox, would see another eighty between them. An outbreak of influenza in March 1837 made them even busier. One day Edward and Lomax saw eighty patients each. They treated influenza with emetics and purgatives of calomel, antimony or jalap, with 'acetate of morphine' for the cough, and demand was

---

182 Steggall, J., *A manual for students preparing for examination at Apothecaries Hall or other medical examinations,* p 465.

183 Moore, J.W., *Eruptive and Continued Fevers,* Dublin, Fannin and Co, 1892, p. 297. Moore notes that there were 98 names for typhus, including Jail Fever, Ship Fever and Irish Ague. Hippocrates used the term 'Typhus' which is derived from the Greek for 'smoke, mist or fog', and refers to the confusion of mind experienced by sufferers.

so heavy that stocks of medicine ran out. Some more seriously ill patients 'needed the lancet', that is, blood-letting. Such was the faith of medical men of the time in bleeding that one of Edward's patients had 'lost upwards of 60 oz'[184] though he would have done better to keep it. Despite this potentially harmful and now long-abandoned treatment, Edward was glad to report that no patient died. Benjamin had influenza in London, and at home Edward, his mother Elizabeth and sister Betsey all suffered from it, though 'Fanny escaped'.

There were many difficult midwifery cases, including prolonged and obstructed labours with stillborn babies to the distress of all concerned. Edward did not tell his brother about one unsuccessful medical case: in 1835 he was called to see Adelaide Darby's aunt, Ann Sorton whose daughter Maria married Richard Darby, who was suffering from pneumonia.[185] He bled her, as conventional treatment required but, according to Adelaide, 'it was not thought that [he] had healed her judiciously'. Mr Webb of Wellington was therefore called and said that, although the patient was very weak, the only hope was to bleed her further, and despite his having 'expressed little hope that her strength would be sufficient to rally after it,' more blood was taken. She died a few hours later. Edward's conservative approach was probably the better one and it seems unjust that he should be disparaged for his caution and that Webb should be applauded for hastening the patient's demise.

Edward was fortunate in having a competent assistant in Lomax, who, during the typhus and influenza epidemics, had 'conducted himself throughout this arduous time with such diligence and satisfaction to the patients generally as to merit my warmest approbation'. Yet Lomax's tenure in the practice was by no means secure. In 1836, a certain Mrs Knight told Edward that Lomax was 'a regular admirer of her daughter' though he was in no position to marry even if he wished

---

184   60 fluid ounces is 3 pints, or nearly 2 litres.

185   Thomas, Emyr, (ed.), *The Private Journal of Adelaide Darby of Coalbrookdale*, p. 24.

to do so. Edward wrote 'it is of course not pleasant, but as he conducts himself very well I wink at it, otherwise I should dismiss him'. Such were the insecurities of Nineteenth-Century life. It was just as well that Lomax was so competent because, with all the hard work, Edward was ill himself and needed reliable help. If Lomax had to leave, or if Edward became more seriously ill, he would need Benjamin's help. He told his brother:

> Should my health continue as at present I am afraid it will be necessary for you to come home, I shall not call upon you if I can avoid it but it may be as well to prepare for it.[186]

The unusually short letter ended:

> I feel so unwell and fatigued with writing that I must conclude'
> I am dear Benjamin,
> Y^r Aff^e brother, E. Edwards

The stress of the typhus and influenza epidemics of 1836 and the recurrence of influenza in the following winter had taken its toll on Edward, the family bread-winner. But by March 1837 he was feeling better: 'after dragging myself through the winter with great difficulty from rheumatism I have nearly regained my health'. Edward was therefore content for his brother to stay in London, take his examinations and return to the practice as a qualified doctor. But it seemed that Benjamin had other ideas — to come home for the summer and defer his exams for a year. Was he really committed to the life of a general practitioner in what was becoming an industrial backwater? Edward had his doubts.

---

[186] SA, 1987/56/7, Letter, Edward to Benjamin.

Chapter 9

Reform and Partnership

As Edward's health improved, Benjamin was able to continue his studies but he may have found life in London more challenging and his studies more complex than his brother had done twenty years before. Big changes were occurring in the structure of medical education. Increasing knowledge and changing practices demanded a new curriculum which would be more suitable to a university than to the disparate private schools and independent teachers of the past. Moves were afoot to found such a university in London which, if Benjamin took notice, may have bewildered the young man from distant Shropshire. Furthermore, the affair of Thomas Smith and the Apothecaries' Society may have led Benjamin to doubt his ability when it came to being examined himself or even to doubt whether he really wanted to be a doctor at all. Although Edward had said 'a man must make his business his amusement', Benjamin may have feared he would not find the medical business as 'amusing' as his brother did.

Even in Edward's time there was much to be learned, as shown by the following statements from one of the more popular student books, the 1823 edition of Steggal's *Manual for Students*, which indicate the increase in scientific knowledge required of students since Benjamin Wright's time:

- Animal and vegetable bodies are formed by a series of compounds, named proximate principals [and consist of] four elements, viz. oxygen, hydrogen, carbon and nitrogen.

- Organic bodies are distinguished by the impossibility of imitating them by the chemical art.

- Composition of citric acid is 2 parts hydrogen, 4 oxygen, 4 carbon, 2 water

- Morphia is the alkaline principal of opium [and is a combination of] meconic acid, codeia, narcotine, resin &c, and may be procured by macerating opium in water.

- Pancreatic juice resembles saliva and contains in addition albumen and ozmaome. [It is distinguished] from saliva of the mouth by not containing sulphocyanic acid.

In the fifteen years between Edward taking the LSA and Benjamin starting his studies there had been even greater progress in medical science, especially in chemistry. In clinical medicine, diseases were no longer described loosely as 'fever' or 'dyspepsia', but were being classified and distinguished from one another, which made accurate diagnosis increasingly important.

This description of the symptoms of measles from Steggal's student text-book is not unlike one that might be found today:

> *Symptoms:* Pyrexia, cough, hoarseness, dyspnoea, wheezing, sneezing, coryza and drowsiness. On about the fourth day an eruption of dingy red prominent spots ... show themselves on the face and neck and gradually spread over the body.[187]

Whether or not Benjamin had misgivings about his studies, on 13 September 1838 he was examined for the LSA by Mr Wheeler and 'approved',[188] and was also successful in the membership examination

---

187 Steggall, John, *A manual for students preparing for examination at Apothecaries Hall or other medical examinations,* 1838.

188 Mrs J. Payne, Archivist at Society of Apothecaries, personal communication 21 Mar 2011.

for the Royal College of Surgeons (MRCS). He then returned to the family medical business in Coalbrookdale and, having thus 'passed the College and Hall', could legitimately call himself 'Physician and Surgeon'. At this point the correspondence between the brothers in London and Shropshire ends and, with it, nearly all accounts of their practice. Some mysteries about Benjamin's commitment remain, however, that suggest that he was not as dedicated to the work as his brother had hoped.

While Benjamin was thus completing his studies, the necessary reform of medical education and the legal status of the profession began in earnest. Contributions to the debate took place not just in London but all over the country, in some of which Edward made his democratic contribution. There were four strands to these reforms:

- The foundation of medical faculties in new universities in London and elsewhere.

- The enquiry into medical education by a Parliamentary Select Committee.

- The formation of a professional body for all doctors, in contrast to the self-interested medical corporations.

- The Medical Act of 1858.

Proposals for a new university in London began in 1825, when a group of eminent people under the leadership of Dr George Birkbeck[189]

---

189 George Birkbeck (1776-1841) was a Quaker from Settle, Yorkshire. He was an eminent physician in London who was also a pioneer in education, particularly in creating the Society for the Diffusion of Useful Knowledge and the Mechanics Institution to educate the working classes. He was a prime mover in the foundation of London University, and gave his name to one of its institutions, Birkbeck College. ONB, online edition, accessed 1 Jun 2013

and Henry Brougham MP[190] proposed the foundation of a non-sectarian college for students excluded from Oxford and Cambridge because they were not members of the Church of England. Eight acres of land were acquired in Bloomsbury for the new University College, which took its first students in 1828.[191] At first medical subjects were taught in a house in Gower Street, and clinical experience was available in a new dispensary in Euston Square associated with the College. In-patient wards were added to the Dispensary in 1837, which later became University College Hospital and incorporated the Gower Street medical school.

Because the Anglican establishment disapproved of the non-conformist principles of the Bloomsbury venture a rival institution was founded to ensure that its religious beliefs were maintained in university education. Under the patronage of King George IV and situated next to Somerset House in the Strand, it was named King's College. It too had a medical school associated with a new hospital. Though King's and University Colleges were separate institutions, in 1837 both became parts of the new University of London under a charter which gave it the right to award degrees, including medical degrees. The University of London was thus based on a collegiate system, like that of Cambridge University, which in due course included the medical schools of The London, Guy's, St Thomas's, Middlesex, King's and St Bartholomew's hospitals. Medical schools were subsequently founded at other London hospitals, and new universities were created

---

190 Henry, First Baron Brougham and Vaux (1778-1868) was Lord Chancellor and a great supporter of both the Parliamentary Reform Act and the Poor Law Amendment Act. His Scottish education influenced him in his contribution to the foundation of London University as a non-sectarian institution open to all. His influence in parliament was vital in securing its charter in 1835. ONB, online edition, accessed 1 Jun 2013.

191 Harte, N., *The University of London, 1836-1986,* London, The Athlone Press, 1986, pp 68-74.

in cities such as Bristol, Birmingham and Manchester. As the medical schools in the various London hospitals were merged into the University, the unregulated miscellany of apprenticeships, private schools and clinical experience ceased to exist. The Apothecaries Society continued to offer an examination for the LSA but never developed any teaching facilities.

The second element of medical reform was the Parliamentary Select Committee's enquiry into medical education. Before the new university was established the disparate elements of medical teaching were unregulated, so, in 1834, Parliament appointed a Select Committee to examine the whole question of medical education.[192] Sir Henry Halford, President of the Royal College of Physicians (RCP), told the committee that for many years it had been his college's policy to prevent surgeons and apothecaries from practising as physicians. He acknowledged that the public had recently shown 'a great tendency' to employ general practitioners, many of whom had 'acquired great credit with the public without being physicians'. But apothecaries and surgeons practised manual crafts including midwifery whereas the practice of physic was an intellectual one. Allowing manual craftsmen to be licentiates of the College would 'throw discredit' on its fellows who had been educated at university to 'improve their minds in literary and scientific acquirements'. Halford insisted that the three 'branches of the healing art' should remain distinct for the 'good of science', therefore a candidate for the licence of the College must 'disenfranchise himself from any community that is not strictly medical', by which he meant the corporations of the Surgeons and the Apothecaries. Yet when asked if he approved of the system whereby apothecaries were only allowed to charge for medicines but not for their advice or attendance he replied 'No, I set my face very much against it. I had rather they were paid for their trouble', which was somewhat at variance with his objection to apothecaries acting as physicians.

---

192 Parliamentary Select Committee on Medical Education, 1834.

Another eminent witness was Dr Neil Arnott, one of the great advocates of medical reform. He had paid thirty guineas to be examined for membership of the Royal College of Surgeons (RCS) and had purchased his MD from Marischal College in Aberdeen without examination. To extend his credentials he sought to become a licentiate of the RCP but, under the laws of the college, he was not allowed to be both physician *and* surgeon so he renounced his membership of the RCS which cost him twenty guineas. He said the rules of the RCP had originally been designed to prevent 'ignorant men and quacks' from practising as physicians but now they were used to prevent apothecaries behaving like physicians in order to 'protect the personal advantage of members and the corporate advantage of the College'. Yet apothecaries had improved their standards so much that they were even attracting men from Oxford and Cambridge and had so 'raised the character of that class' that there were now more apothecaries and fewer physicians than previously. In a forthright criticism of the RCP he said the college was not 'using its authority to raise the character of the profession and increase efficiency', because:

> It had been perverted to other purposes and produced the effect of throwing nineteen-twentieths of the whole medical practice of the country ... into the hands of persons not physicians, although the College was created to embrace the whole.

Arnott said this acrimonious policy had even included attempts to imprison transgressors, so that, instead of bringing surgeons and physicians together, they had insulted honourable men and prevented useful dialogue. His thirty-minute oral examination for the license of the College had been so inadequate that an ignorant person could have passed if asked something he happened to know about, yet a competent person might fail if a few gaps in his knowledge were exposed. He thought there ought to be some body (but not the RCP) consisting of the best medical men in London, including surgeons, with the power to examine all branches of medicine together and grant degrees. There should be no distinction between the various sections of the profession because 'every medical man should be a completely educated man'. His preferred curriculum for all medical students would consist of a complete general education, preliminary studies of physics, chemistry, physiology and psychology or 'philosophy of mind', followed by clinical studies. Doctors should know one classical language, but not waste seven years acquiring a broad classical education. His views on whether general practitioners should be remunerated only by charging for medicines were even more strongly worded than Halford's. He said it was:

> ... a very bad system. It leads to a very complicated system of prescription, and renders very remarkable the form and bulk of medicines the English people swallow. I would give doctors a legal claim to recover [fees] for attendance, medicine or both.

Many witnesses agreed that the out-dated tripartite system should be abandoned, and a new curriculum for students should be predominately medical. The Select Committee's report advocated a system which became the basis of the medical curriculum for more than a hundred years. Benjamin arrived in London just as the new institutions were being opened so could have enrolled as a student of London University but, like his brother before him, he arranged his own curriculum of private lectures and clinical experience to which he added occasional lectures at King's College. The Edwards may not yet have realised the significance of the new university, or perhaps the family's caution in the expenditure of that rare commodity, money, made them choose the familiar path.

In the third element of reform, the voice of provincial practitioners began to be heard again as well as those of the unrepresentative Royal Colleges and Apothecaries' Society. In 1794, apothecaries had met at the Crown and Anchor to demand protection against untrained competitors; in 1802 they protested against the imposition of tax on medicines; in 1814-15 they demanded commercial protection through the Apothecaries Act. All these demands for democratic representation had failed. The mood in the medical profession now resembled that in politics in demanding democratic representation. The Great Reform and Municipal Corporations Acts reduced though did not yet eliminate the oligarcy of political patronage and the self-perpetuating magistracy. The powerful Royal Colleges and the Apothecaries Society began to appear like medical rotten boroughs and the democratic tide was rising so that, Canute-like, it could no longer be resisted by those institutions.

The medical profession had become seriously overcrowded with tens of thousands of doctors who had qualified by LSA or MRCS, but there was still no way for the public to distinguish them from unqualified pretenders. It was not necessary to have had any medical education or to have passed an examination to set up as a 'surgeon' or 'druggist' and many people of dubious reliability offered their services and cures to a gullible public. Doctors who had taken the 'College and Hall' examinations could style themselves 'Physician and Surgeon' but, although they clamoured for protection from untrained rivals, they had no central body to argue their case or represent it to parliament. The only organisations that could do so were the Royal Colleges and the Society of Apothecaries, none of which were concerned with the thousands of general practitioners. A more broadly based system of representation was necessary.

As noted in Chapter 7, the Provincial Medical and Surgical Association (PMSA) was founded in 1832 and was open to every qualified medical and surgical practitioner in Britain, and it was run on democratic lines with all members having the right to vote. Because of restrictions in postage and travel, national events were difficult to advertise effectively — the reach of journals like *The Lancet* was limited and newspapers mostly reported local events. As these limitations were overcome a network of PMSA branches was formed that gave ordinary practitioners a voice in the development of their own profession. In June 1838 the *Salopian Journal* reported that 'about 50 gentlemen of the profession' met at the Lion Hotel in Shrewsbury to form the Shropshire and North Wales Branch of the [Provincial Medical and Surgical] Association.[193] Edward was probably one of those '50 gentlemen', and he certainly attended subsequent meetings. Among the Shropshire branch's early concerns were the low remuneration of Union medical officers and the failure of the Apothecaries Act to protect qualified doctors from unfair competition. Concerns of this kind were debated at local and national meetings and reported in articles and correspondence in *The Lancet* and the new *Journal of the PMSA*, which later became *The British Medical Journal.*

Although general practitioners who had passed the examination of the Royal College of Surgeons and paid their fees felt very strongly that the college should represent its provincial as well as its metropolitan members, the College continued to concern itself only with London surgeons. A vigorous but unsuccessful campaign for representation of provincial doctors was mounted by members of the Shropshire Branch of the PMSA, which earned them the title of 'The Spirited Surgeons of Shropshire' in *The Lancet*.[194] A more direct approach was the four-man delegation that gave evidence to the Parliamentary Select Committee on Medical Registration in 1847. By this time proposals for a Register of qualified doctors were being discussed and would eventually form an important part of the 1858 Medical Act.

---

193 'Provincial Medical and Surgical Association, Shropshire and North Wales Branch', *Salopian Journal*, 20 Jun 1838.

194 *The Lancet*, 1, 1845, p. 464.

The fourth element of the reform was the prolonged campaign by the PMSA and, later, the BMA for legislation to regulate the profession. Democratically convened branches debated the issue and presented petitions to supportive Members of Parliament. After nineteen fruitless parliamentary bills, the campaign succeeded in achieving legal recognition of the profession and protection from unqualified competitors with the passing of the Medical Act in 1858. This created the 'General Council of Medical Education and Registration', now known as the General Medical Council (GMC), which was given the two major responsibilities that its name implies. Under 'Registration' the GMC was required to compile the *Medical Register*, a list of all qualified doctors that would distinguish them from untrained pretenders to medical skills. Doctors already in practice could enter their names on the Register without further examination but, to be eligible, new doctors would have to pass a university medical degree examination or the LSA. Anyone practising as a doctor without registering, or while being ineligible to do so, would render himself liable to prosecution. Under 'Education' the GMC determined the medical curriculum and authorised the final examinations of medical schools. As a result, all medical students would follow the same curriculum and demonstrate their competence to the same standard whether they intended to practise as physician, surgeon or general practitioner. The Medical Act's great achievements were to unify the profession, to ensure that educational standards were consistent and to enable the public to identify practitioners who were properly qualified. Despite its lengthy gestation it was brought about by democratic processes within both the profession and parliament and it remains the regulatory basis of the profession today. Reform of the medical profession had been accomplished: there was a unified system of training at university level; all students studied the same course whatever their intended future as physician or surgeon; duly qualified doctors were distinguishable from others by the Medical

Register; and there was a professional association, the BMA, widely supported and democratically constituted. There was no place for incompetent or dangerous quacks and charlatans.

This diversion into the story of medical reform may have caused the reader temporarily to lose sight of Edward and Benjamin Edwards in their Coalbrookdale practice. The brothers would have followed the progress of the reform campaign through the weekly *Journal of the PMSA* which reported both scientific and medico-political matters. Although the prosperity of Coalbrookdale was in decline, the spark of genius and innovation that began in the Dale became a fire that spread all over Britain. Heavy industries developed in Wolverhampton, Manchester, Newcastle-on-Tyne and elsewhere as Britain was transformed into a manufacturing powerhouse. In 1851, six million people were able to see the produce of the nation and its empire at the Great Exhibition at the Crystal Palace in London, a migration made possible by the new railways. Huge bridges of iron were built that made the modest Iron Bridge look small, and enormous machines produced myriad goods to satisfy the demands of a growing middle class. Iron ships propelled by vast steam engines were built, the most amazing of which was Isambard Kingdom Brunel's 19,000 ton *Great Eastern* that enabled unprecedented transport of passengers and goods across the globe. The British Empire expanded until 'the sun never set upon it' and made Britain the richest nation in the world — though the price was paid by the workers and their families, whose working conditions and wretchedly crowded housing brought new medical challenges of industrial disease and hideous epidemics. By the middle of the Nineteenth Century, Britain was totally changed from that of Benjamin Wright and William Edwards in the tiny industrial enclave of Coalbrookdale where the first iron bridge and the first iron boat had been built and the first steam locomotive developed.

Although the Dale's industrial pre-eminence declined in the early Nineteenth Century, the Coalbrookdale Company took a new direction under Francis Darby by developing the artistic and architectural uses of iron.[195] It was in this ever-changing industrial environment that Edward and Benjamin practised in partnership from 1840 onwards. However, despite the extraordinary progress in industry and science, including some aspects of medicine, there were still few effective treatments for disease. Even where progress had been made, as in smallpox vaccination, Edward doubted its benefits. In 1838 he wrote to Benjamin, 'There is a great quantity of Small Pox. I think now that the Cow Pock [vaccine] is of little value, what is the opinion of it in London?' Benjamin's reply, if there was one, has been lost but, since then, vaccination has rid the world of that horrid disease. In practice, doctors like Edward and Benjamin were able to do little more for their patients than their fathers and grandfathers had done. Almost none of the procedures we take for granted today were available to them and, although cholera, typhus and typhoid became less frequent, they could not be cured. Mines and foundries claimed their victims from accident and diseases that are now preventable and the catch-all diagnosis of 'consumption' still claimed its victims by the thousand.

In one way the work of the general practitioner in Edward and Benjamin's day was similar to that of their professional successors in recent times, in that they were easily accessible because they lived amongst their patients in the community, yet in others it was totally different.[196] Although there were charity-based hospitals, only a tiny minority of patients were treated in them. By the end of the Nineteenth Century many local communities had 'cottage' hospitals, staffed by general practitioners, but there were none near Coalbrookdale until

---

195 Raistrick, A., *Dynasty of Ironfounders: the Darbys of Coalbrookdale*, p. 261-2.

196 In the last few years there have been changes to NHS contracts for GPs that have reduced their twenty-four-hour responsibilities but other activities have increased, especially the management of chronic disease. The author is speaking more of his own experience as a late-Twentieth-Century GP, whose early years seem in retrospect to be more like the Edwards's era than the present (2014).

1902 when one was built in Broseley. A quarryman or farmer who broke a leg would do better to rest at home with his limb splinted than to be carried bumpily in a horse-drawn cart along ten or twenty miles of pot-holed roads to a hospital. And an elderly woman with pneumonia would do better to stay in her own bed to be nursed by relatives than go to hospital where she might catch typhus or dysentery from her fellow patients. Whether a patient stayed at home or went to hospital she might be too drastically bled, like Ann Sorton. Apart from smallpox vaccination there were no immunisations to prevent diseases nor antibiotics to cure infections. Indeed, bacteria and viruses had yet to be discovered. The mid-Nineteenth-Century general practitioner was not only the first line of defence but, in many cases, the last one too.

Some indication of the conditions that Edward and Benjamin might have treated can be seen in the death rates between 1848 and 1872, about the time of their partnership in Coalbrookdale.[197] At that time the death rate was 45,000 per million in England and Wales in a population of about 18 million. Of the 800,000 deaths a year, thirty percent (about 270,000) were caused by infectious diseases, of which one third were tuberculosis. Other deadly infections were scarlet fever and diphtheria, which were not distinguishable from each other at the time (45,000), whooping cough (18,000) and measles (14,000), all of which mostly affected children. Heart attacks and other diseases of the circulation caused 40,000 deaths, and diseases of the nervous system, such as strokes, about 90,000; cancer accounted for less than 4,000 deaths; diabetes accounted for a few hundred, though without modern diagnostic tests it may well have been misdiagnosed as consumption or another wasting disease. Deaths from epidemic infectious disease are now uncommon in Britain and our longer lives are more likely to end with heart disease or cancer.

The diseases that Edward and Benjamin were called upon to treat

---

[197] Charlton, John, and Murphy, Mike, *The Health of Adult Britain, 1841-1994*, pp 27 and 32-36.

ranged from the trivial to the life-threatening or fatal. What could they do when faced with intractable problems, without the modern tools to investigate and diagnose them accurately and with no specific treatments when diagnosed? Their tools were their hands, eyes and ears, the pocket-watch and that newly-invented gadget the stethoscope.[198] They lived at a time in which the nature of diseases was being explored and classified and their modes of transmission understood, but before the means to cure them were developed. Yet two major advances did occur in their lifetime: one was the discovery of anaesthesia in the 1840s, which could make surgery and childbirth painless, the other was improved hygiene through supply of clean water and removal of sewage, though neither of these developments was for general practitioners to implement. The antiseptic technique introduced by Joseph Lister in 1865, which made surgery safer, was too late for the Edwards brothers. In fact there was little improvement in what general practitioners could do for their patients and, in retrospect, it is disappointing that the only personal recollection of the brothers' practice seems somewhat unfair. It comes from the diary of Charles Peskin (1862-1948) who lived in the Dale, but as the diary only begins in 1876 it is very late in Edward and Benjamin's time as the Coalbrookdale doctors. Charles Peskin said:

> They were doctors of the old school, and believed in cupping, bleeding and leeching, and when a club or panel patient (as a person was known who was away from work and receiving treatment) came to the Doctors for treatment they were invariably given a couple of ounces of Epsom Salts and told to come back later.[199]

---

198 Watches with reliable second hands for counting the pulse rate came into use in the early Nineteenth Century. Before then, the pulse was described as either 'rapid' or 'slow' but the actual rate per minute was not counted.

199 Jones, Ken, *Pitmen, Poachers and Preachers: Life and the Poor Law in the Madeley Union of Parishes, 1700-1930,* Ludlow, The Dog Rose Press, 2009, p.241.

This cursory mention of the doctors probably reflects more on the treatments then available than the qualities of the doctors themselves. Though powerless to intervene in their patients' illnesses, there was much else to do: a sympathetic hearing, kind words in distress or emotional support when a patient, perhaps a young child, was dying. These are important aspects of good medical care even now, and essential when there is no cure.

Two other anecdotes illustrate the doctors' activities and reveal something of their different characters. The first is the case of William Morgan who suffered a blow on the side of his head.[200] Edward described a large wound and 'considerable fracture', and said the patient was slightly delirious. He said there had been 'no pain, the pulse was not disturbed, pupils not affected, and senses perfect', and treated the injury as 'a common wound'. Two days later he was called again because Morgan had fainted, though he recovered quickly. Swelling of the wound caused several pieces of bone to protrude, which Edward removed. While he was doing this, the patient 'sat up perfectly sensible and supported his head with his elbows resting on the bedstead, [and the operation] was attended with neither good nor ill consequences'. Edward said his patient 'asked very calmly if I thought he would recover' and, the next day, he was sitting up 'perfectly sensible' while the doctor was there. The following day, however, 'the brain rose through the wound and he died ten days later'. Edward's clinical examination was careful and correct, noting his patient's level of consciousness and the state of the pulse and pupils. If only he had known about germs and infection: if only he had not removed the bits of bone; if only antibiotics, X rays and MRI scans had been available … but Edward was a child of his time and could not foresee those marvellous things that, one day, would help to cure such unfortunate people as William Morgan.

The other anecdote has echoes of that 'want of government' in Benjamin's behaviour which Edward had commented upon twenty-five years earlier. George Bailey, a young millwright, was repairing a

---

200 SA, 1987/56/5, Letter, Edward to Benjamin

large shearing machine in a pit when a heavy piece of metal fell on him 'crushing his head against the top of the ditch in a frightful manner'.[201] A messenger was sent to find a doctor urgently and Mr Soames, who lived nearby, attended the scene. He found there was nothing he could do to save the young man but did arrange for him to be carried home (not to hospital) and stayed to comfort the victim's sister and widowed mother. When he heard that the family were patients of the Edwards brothers, who were also the works doctors, Soames sent a message asking one of them to come immediately. The messenger found Benjamin, who was out visiting patients, but he refused to help saying that he would not do so as long as Mr Soames was there. Despite repeated requests, Benjamin adamantly refused to visit the injured man and his grieving relatives. Later in the day yet another messenger found Edward, who according to the report in the *Wellington Journal*:

> ... appeared very indignant at the conduct of his brother and immediately went and met with Mr Soames at the poor man's residence. It need hardly be said that nothing could be done to alleviate his suffering.

Because George Bailey died following an accident, an inquest was held (at the Foresters' Arms, not the Coroner's Court). The jury reached a verdict of accidental death to which they added the following comment:

> The jury desire to express their strong disapprobation of the conduct and the behaviour of Mr B. Edwards in refusing to attend or see the deceased on being repeatedly requested so to do, and at the same time giving no other reason than that another medical man had previously been in attendance on him'.

---

201   *Wellington Journal*, 18 May 1861, Fatal Accident at the Iron Works: strange behaviour of a medical attendant.

We do not know what was said between Edward and Benjamin that evening but the reader may imagine its likely tone. It may be supposed that Benjamin's reasoning arose from a vague ethical idea that a doctor should not interfere with another doctor's treatment, though in such circumstances this convention could reasonably have been disregarded. What made Benjamin behave in this seemingly heartless way? There has long been an understanding that doctors do not offer their services to patients who are under the care of another doctor, but that was not the situation here. Mr Soames had been called in a dire emergency and could hardly refuse to attend, but was ready to leave as soon as the patient's usual doctor could be found. Thomas Percival's *Medical Ethics*[202] specifically states that a doctor may see a patient of another if the regular doctor is unavailable, and take appropriate action until the usual one returns. Admittedly, Percival's book had been published sixty years earlier but the common sense advice would seem to hold good. Another widely respected book on medical ethics, published shortly after this incident by the Shropshire physician Jukes de Styrap, is clear:

> The right of a patient to change or to discard his medical adviser is unquestionable ... [but] a medical practitioner is justly entitled to expect that he shall not without cause and reasonable courtesy and explanation be superseded in attendance on a case.[203]

So why did Benjamin refuse to comfort the injured man, his sickly mother (who was probably under his care at that very time) and his dependent sister? Was it a misunderstanding of the proper relationship between competing colleagues? Was he afraid he could not cope with such a demanding case? Or was he horrified by injury, pain and death?

---

202 Percival, Thomas, *Medical Ethics,* London, 1803, p. 47.

203 Styrap, Jukes de, *A Code of Medical Ethics,* London, H. K. Lewis, 4th ed., 1895, p. 47.

No such sensitivities prevented his brother Edward from answering the call when he belatedly heard of the tragedy. There is another possibility which throws doubt on Benjamin's commitment to his profession. The accident that killed George Bailey occurred only three years after the 1858 Medical Act, which required all duly qualified medical practitioners to enter their names on the Medical Register. Benjamin was eligible to do so but his name does not appear in the first Register of 1859 or any other Register for the next ten years. The need to register cannot have escaped him because Edward entered his own name, and any doctors who were eligible but failed to do so were under pressure from colleagues to comply with the law. In many places, including Shropshire, 'Medico-Ethical Associations' were formed to ensure compliance and to arrange for the entries of any ineligible men who had succeeded in registering to be erased. The whole point of the Medical Act was to prevent unqualified and unregistered people from practising — and by continuing to do so without registering Benjamin was flouting the law. We cannot know 150 years later why Benjamin did not register and it would be unfair to castigate him without knowing his reasons.

At the time of the George Bailey affair sixty-two-year-old Edward may have been reducing his workload, but at forty-four Benjamin would still have to earn his living despite a change in his social status. Whereas their apothecary father and grandfather had been in trade, Edward and Benjamin were now members of the professional middle class. Furthermore they had inherited money which enabled them to move up another rung on the social ladder. They had become 'gentry'.

Chapter 10

Finale

Thirty years of debate within the profession and parliament culminated in the Medical Act of 1858. It created a register of all doctors who had passed a test of competence to practise, established the legal definition of the profession and made it illegal to practise if unqualified and unregistered. Edward was eligible to register because not only had he passed the LSA and MRCS, but was already in practice, so he could call himself a 'registered medical practitioner', rather than 'apothecary' or 'surgeon'. Although the word 'doctor' had long been used to describe the role of such a person it was not yet used as a title or prefix to a name except by those physicians who had a university doctorate.[204] Edward therefore remained plain 'Mr' Edwards. Both Edward and Benjamin are described in the censuses of 1861 and 1871 as 'medical practitioners' without the word 'registered'. In fact Benjamin never registered, as he should have done while continuing to practise. He is listed in the 1871 census as 'MRCS and licensed apothecary *not practising*, though he was then only fifty-four years old. By 1881 he is listed as 'retired doctor'.

The 1850s brought changes to the family that were variously sad and bountiful. In 1851 there were seven people living at Rose Hill, namely William's seventy-nine-year-old widow Elizabeth, Betsey (fifty-three), Edward (fifty-two), Fanny (forty-three) and Benjamin (thirty-five) as well as their two servants, the thirty-year-old cook Emma Reynolds and Sarah Bird the nineteen-year-old maid. It was a large household for a small house. Although there is no record of life at Rose Hill after

---

204 The use of the prefix 'Dr' before a practitioner's name did not become usual until the end of the 19th Century. General practitioners retained the prefix 'Mr', as did surgeons who did not usually have a university doctorate.

FINALE

Benjamin's return from London, the earlier letters suggest they were a warm and affectionate family with musical interests and many contacts with their cousins and others in the Dale. Elizabeth passed away on 25th January 1855, at the commendably old age of eighty-three after twenty-seven years of widowhood. The winter of 1855 was very cold with frequent heavy snow which perhaps hastened her demise. Her death was reported in *Eddowes Journal* of 31st January:

> 25th January, after a long and painful illness borne with pious resignation in her 84th year, Elizabeth, relict of the late William Edwards, Esq, surgeon, deeply lamented.

She was not buried with her husband at Malinslee but at the newly-consecrated Holy Trinity Church in Coalbrookdale. Adelaide Darby briefly noted Elizabeth's death in her diary on 28th January: 'old Mrs Edwards is dead'. Adelaide had spent much of February and March in London but, on her return to Coalbrookdale, she called on Betsey and Fanny to express her condolences.[205] The Darbys and Edwards were neighbours although not quite social equals, even though the Darbys were descended from artisan smiths and brass-founders and the Edwards from tradesmen apothecaries. There is a hint of the social difference between them at this time in Adelaide's diary: she refers to her 'drawing room' but, of the Edwards, to their 'parlour'.

The family were still mourning the loss of their mother when sorrow struck again. On 7th June their uncle Peter Wright died at the age of seventy-nine and was laid to rest in a plot near his sister Elizabeth's grave at Holy Trinity. Worse was to follow because, within weeks, Fanny fell ill and, on 18th August, she died, aged only forty-seven. Within eight months Betsey, Edward and Benjamin had lost their

---

205 Thomas, E. (ed.), *The Private Journal of Adelaide Darby of Coalbrookdale, from 1833 to 1861,* 14 April 1855.

mother, uncle and sister. Years before, in 1827 when she was only twenty years old, Fanny had been gravely ill with typhus and may have been something of an invalid since then, but that would not account for the suddenness of her death which was possibly due smallpox, pneumonia or a sudden complication of tuberculosis. Of William and Elizabeth's four daughters only Betsey, the oldest, was still alive and she remained at Rose Hill with Edward and Benjamin.

Then an alteration in their financial affairs completely changed their circumstances.

Earlier generations of the family had owned land in Shropshire and later in Norfolk and Lincolnshire. Their estates, or the capital from their sale, had been passed down the generations and in due course some of this wealth had come to William's older brother Richard, then living in London. When he died in 1835 without children the inheritance was shared with his nephews in Coalbrookdale and their cousin, another William Edwards, who lived at Spalding in Lincolnshire. Edward attended his uncle's funeral in London, and then went to Spalding to meet his cousin who was an executor to Richard's will jointly with Edward. He wrote to his mother from Spalding:

> My uncle was interred the evening of Friday & I left London at six o'clock & arrived in Spalding on Saturday morning at Breakfast. Unfortunately Mr Edwards is from home but I expect to meet him on the road. I have been able to accomplish with his son Mr Wm Edwards principally what I wanted & shall leave the will with them to prove &c &c. Mr Edwards's family are delightfully happy and it is a great pleasure to meet such relatives who have been so little known to us — there is a great Family resemblance.[206]

---

206 SA, 1987/56/30, Letter, Edward at Spalding to Elizabeth: no date.

Legal matters are not remarkable for the rapidity of their execution and, although William Edwards was an attorney, very little happened for two years. Then, in December 1836, Edward wrote to Benjamin in a tone of eager anticipation, saying:

> I have received intelligence from Spalding & a promise of the Account of the Norfolk property at Xmas when I shall expect a considerable remittance.[207]

Three months later Edward had still heard nothing, let alone received his 'remittance'. Another two years went by until in 1838 an exasperated Edward again wrote to his brother:

> I have not heard from Spalding & begin to feel anxious, they seem as tardy as ever. If you can learn when Mr J. [who is unidentified] writes home it would be as well to hint to him that I am desirous of hearing from them.[208]

The favourable impression his cousins had made at first acquaintance now seemed to be fading.

Eventually the long-awaited 'considerable remittance' did arrive and it enabled Edward to purchase the freehold of Rose Hill, which provided a secure home for the family and especially for Betsey if she were to outlive her brothers. He also invested in other property, including his uncle Peter Wright's house at Greenbank, built by Peter's father Benjamin on land leased from the Earl of Craven for a sixty-three-year term that happened to expire just at the time of Peter's death. Edward was thus able to purchase the freehold of house

---

[207] SA, 1987/56/9, Letter, Edward to Benjamin, 18 Dec. 1836.

[208] SA, 1987/56/11, Letter, Edward to Benjamin, 7 Apr. 1838.

and land.[209] However, he and Betsey continued to live at Rose Hill from where the medical practice was still conducted. Edward also acquired other property in the area — farmland formerly known as The Woodlands and buildings and gardens in Holloway Lane in the parish of Dawley, and land called 'The Old Incline' which he bought from the Coalbrookdale Company.

Benjamin bought a house of his own at Stoney Hill, a mile or so away on the road to Lightmoor. That property, which is now buried under the refuse of the citizens of Telford, consisted of a substantial dwelling house and gardens, together with several cottages occupied by tenants. At some time in the 1860s, when he was in his forties, Benjamin set up home there with a housekeeper, the widow Sarah Evans who was eleven years younger than him. It would be prying into their privacy to read too much into the meaning of the word 'housekeeper' but, as Benjamin was very generous to her in his will, the reader may like to speculate on the degree of intimacy in their relationship in those strict Victorian days. Sometime in the 1860s, Benjamin gave up medical work to become a gentleman of independent means, with a household consisting of his housekeeper, the sixty-three-year-old cook, Martha Evans, and a nineteen-year old maid, Mary Hart.

Edward's long and hard-working life came to an end on 17th October 1870. His death was announced to the profession in *The Medical Times and Gazette*:

> Deaths: Edward Edwards, Surgeon, Coalbrookdale, Salop, on October 17th, aged 72.[210]

Under his will the family home at Rose Hill and most of his property, money and domestic goods were left to Betsey for the rest

---

209 SA, 1987/28/24, Contained in recital of will of Benjamin Wright.
210 *Medical Times and Gazette*, 1872, Vol 2, p492.

of her lifetime.[211] Greenbank was left to Benjamin but, since he died childless, it was eventually inherited by his cousin William Henry Wright, son of Peter and grandson of the man who had built it nearly eighty years before. Betsey died in 1878 at the age of eighty. Though the oldest of the family, she outlived all her siblings except Benjamin who was eighteen years her junior. She had been Edward's loyal sister and companion for over seventy years and remained single, never having met her 'man possessed of a good fortune who was in need of a wife'. Perhaps her kind of good fortune was to have a dependable brother, Edward, who provided her with a home and left her in comfortable circumstances, socially and financially. She thus fulfilled another of Jane Austen's criteria for a single woman's contentment: that although such a person might be 'a ridiculous disagreeable old maid ... she may be as respectable, sensible and pleasant as anybody else'.[212]

Edward left small legacies to his servants, including nineteen guineas to each of his farm bailiff, his waggoner and his personal servant Edward Johnson, and smaller sums to the female house servants Elizabeth Roberts and Sarah Haines. He bequeathed £50 to his former assistant John Fox who was still living in Coalbrookdale, and of whom he had spoken so highly during the influenza epidemic of 1837. He did not forget some of the less fortunate people he had encountered in his many years as doctor in the Dale, where he had seen at close hand the hardship caused by illness, accident and poverty. He therefore left an endowment of £3,200 to yield an income to buy bread, coals and clothing for poor widows of the district who were members of the Church of England. The beneficiaries were to be selected by the Minister and Churchwardens of Holy Trinity Church from among 'known objects of charity'. A finely engraved and decorated brass memorial near the entrance to the church where Edward worshipped

---

211 SA, 1987/28/17, Will of Edward Edwards.

212 Jane Austen, in *Emma*.

still reminds visitors of his generosity to his less fortunate neighbours.

There was also a bequest of £500 to support the Salop Infirmary which, at this time, was a charity funded entirely by voluntary subscriptions. Patients were admitted on the written recommendation of a subscriber who could recommend one patient at a time for each pound per year subscribed. The bequest was divided between Coalbrookdale church which had the use of half of it and the parishes of Little Wenlock and Doorsley, which had one quarter each. If the bequest yielded, say, 3% per annum this would allow fifteen patients to be admitted, so it was a very valuable asset to the locality. Edward also left £500 to his former pupil, Dr Thomas Banks, and similar sums to his cousin Joseph Yate and other relatives. The whole estate was valued at £10,000, which is roughly equivalent to one million pounds today. It came from assets both earned and inherited which had been managed by a conscientious man — perhaps he shared the financial acumen of his grandfather who had been unofficial banker to the neighbourhood. It was a considerable change of fortune for someone whose family had 'suffered many privations' to enable him to study in London and whose father's overcoat had been 'almost too shabby to wear' as he travelled on his rounds in the bitter cold of winter.

Benjamin lived at Stoney Hill until his death in 1881, which was also recorded in *The Medical Times and Gazette*:

> Deaths: Edwards, Benjamin, MRCS, LAC, at Stoney Hill, Coalbrookdale on October 13th, aged 67.[213]

His estate was valued at over £12,000, and his will suggests that he had amassed a collection of books, prints, pictures and musical instruments (the reader will recall that as a boy he had asked his brother Edward to buy him a fiddle and a gun) as well as a menagerie

---

213 *Medical Times and Gazette*, 1882, Vol 2, p542.

FINALE

of parrots.[214] His major bequest was to his housekeeper Sarah Evans, consisting of £400 for her immediate use and the income from £8,000 in Government Stocks, out of which she was to maintain the house and look after the parrots. She also received the use of the furniture, books, plate, wines, liquors and consumable stores' at Stoney Hill and of the house and its cottages for herself during her lifetime. But she had to 'continue single and unmarried'. The will stipulated that if she were to cohabit, live or lodge with any unmarried male person or take any such unmarried person to live or lodge with her' her income from this bequest would 'absolutely cease'.

Five months before his death Benjamin made a codicil by which the parrots would be Sarah's property only during her lifetime. He must have realised that the birds might outlive their custodian — parrots can live in captivity for more than forty years. After Sarah Evans's death most of the property was to pass to his cousin Joseph Yate of Madeley and thence, eventually, to Arthur Edwards, one of the family's distant cousins in Lincolnshire. There were small bequests of ten shillings a week to some of his cottage tenants but, unlike his brother, he left nothing to the poor and needy of the Dale.

Though Benjamin wanted to be buried in his garden, he was interred beside Fanny, Edward, Betsey and his mother in the churchyard at Holy Trinity, Coalbrookdale, which overlooks the place where they spent their lives. Their graves, which commemorate a family who served the people of the Dale for nearly a hundred years, are surrounded by iron railings that have protected them from changes in the Dale even more far-reaching than those that occurred in their lifetimes.

§

---

214 SA, 1987/28/27, Copy of the Will of Benjamin Edwards.

The view from the churchyard to-day is much the same as it was when William Williams painted it in 1771: the ironmaster's houses and workers' cottages can be glimpsed between the trees on the slopes of the well-wooded valley, with the hills beyond the Severn Gorge in the distance. But the clamour of hammers and forges is heard no more, no barges or trows throng the river and Anna Seward's 'umber'd flames' no longer 'bicker on the hills'. Only a few buildings of the old Coalbrookdale Company remain, now part of the Ironbridge Gorge Museum. The industrial storm has passed, the 'fuliginous' air has cleared and the Dale has regained some of its former tranquillity. The era of Benjamin Wright and his family has come to an end but has left a legacy of its own.

During the lifetimes of the Coalbrookdale doctors the spark of genius that fired the industrial revolution had transformed the world. The use of coke led to the modern iron industry, the first iron bridge and the first iron boat and, for nearly a hundred years, the doctors had been witnesses to that transformation. Benjamin Wright saw the first iron bridge being built, all 379 tons of it; William Edwards must have seen Trevithick's experimental 'locomotive' in action; Edward and Benjamin studied the new sciences of chemistry and physics as part of their medical curriculum. The huge changes in their lifetimes can be illustrated with three examples. A much greater iron bridge now spans the River Forth — one and a half miles long and weighing 58,000 tons; Trevithick's small beginnings developed into thousands of miles of railways, carrying freight and passengers on steam-powered trains; Faraday's experiments with feeble electric currents opened the way to the electric telegraph, lights in streets and houses, power in factories and eventually to radios, mobile phones and computers.

The industrial age brought medical progress in its wake: life expectancy increased; epidemics were controlled; scientific research began to explain the invisible chemical processes in living cells; diseases were described more accurately. At one time apothecaries only kept shops and sold medicines, which they persuaded their patients — and themselves — were effective. As knowledge improved, apothecaries became purely medical men and learned to diagnose illnesses and treat them more rationally, and renamed their shops as 'surgeries'. The clubs of Edward's day that enabled the poor to pay their medical bills became an insurance system based on trades and occupations. These schemes were incorporated into Lloyd George's National Insurance scheme of 1911, until that too was swept away in 1948 with the creation of the National Health Service. It was an evolutionary process, much like that described in 1859 by Charles Darwin in *On the Origin of Species,* in which changes in the environment of a species prompt it to adapt. When the environment of the Dale and the wider world changed, the Coalbrookdale doctors adapted and the new form of 'general practice' survived.

There is still a medical practice in Coalbrookdale. If Edward or Benjamin could visit it today they would surely be astonished by the differences from their own time: bleeding, leeches and 'tonics' have been abandoned; epidemics of smallpox and filth diseases no longer blight the community; diseases can be prevented by immunisation; medicines are specific and effective; crippling arthritis can be relieved by artificial joints ... and much more. But once-rare conditions like cancer, diabetes and heart attacks are now common and new problems of industrial disease and HIV-Aids have arisen. Practices are staffed by receptionists, nurses, midwives, health visitors, physiotherapists and others. Edward and Benjamin (life-long bachelors in a male-dominated age) would surely be surprised to find women among their professional successors. Yet, though astounded by the extent of the change, they could be proud of their legacy: by adapting their thinking and practices to changes in their social and scientific environments they and their contemporaries helped to shape the health-care system of modern Britain.

General practice still faces serious challenges because, as society becomes more mobile and fragmented, so medicine becomes more specialised and the difficulties of the generalist increase. The need for accessible, compassionate and personal doctors is as great as ever and the species that was the Victorian medical practitioner is not extinct. Darwin-like, it has adapted to change. The challenge to general practice today is the same as two centuries ago — adapt, or cease to exist.

Bibliography

Books

Austen, Jane, *Pride and Prejudice* and *Emma*.

Beasley, Henry, *The Book of Prescriptions,* London, John Churchill, 1854.

Chadwick, E., *The Sanitary Condition of the Labouring Population of Great Britain, 1842.* (ed.) Flinn, M.W., Edinburgh University Press, 1965.

Charlton, John and Murphy, Mike, *The Health of Adult Britain, 1841-1994,* London, The Stationery Office, 1997.

Concise Oxford Dictionary of Place-Names, Oxford University Press, 1960.

Fleetwood, John F., *The History of Medicine in Ireland,* Dublin, The Skellig Press, 1983, quoting from *Gilborne's Medical Review,* 1775.

Gatrell, V. A. C., *The Hanging Tree: execution and the English people 1770-1868,* Oxford University Press, 1994.

Gray, E., *Man-midwife: the diary of John Knyveton*, London, Robert Hale Limited, 1944.

Harte, Negley, *The University of London, 1836-1986,* London, The Athlone Press, 1986.

Hodge, J., *Richard Trevithick,* Botley, Oxford, Shire Publications, 1973.

Jones, Ken, *Pitmen, Poachers and Preachers: Life and the Poor Law in the Madeley Union of Parishes, 1700-1930,* Ludlow, The Dog Rose Press, 2009.

Labouchere, Rachel, *Deborah Darby of Coalbrookdale, 1754-1810,* William Session Ltd, York, 1993.

Lawrence, Susan C., *Charitable Knowledge: hospital pupils and practitioners in eighteenth century London,* Cambridge University Press, 1996.

Loudon, Irvine, *Medical Care and the General Practitioner, 1750-1850.* Oxford, The Clarendon Press, 1986.

McMenemey, William H., *The Life and Times of Sir Charles Hastings,* Edinburgh and London, E & S Livingstone, 1959.

Meiklejohn, Andrew, *The Life, Work and Times of Charles Turner Thackrah, 1795-1883,* London, E. & S. Livingstone, 1957.

Moore, John W., *Eruptive and Continued Fevers,* Dublin, Fannin and Co, 1892.

Newman, Charles, *The Evolution of Medical Education in the Nineteenth Century,* Oxford University Press, 1957.

Oxford Dictionary of National Biography, on-line edition.

Pattison, Andrew. *The Darwins of Shrewsbury,* The History Press, Stroud, Gloucestershire, 2009.

Percival, Thomas, *Medical Ethics,* London, 1803.

Plymley, Joseph, *General View of the Agriculture of Shropshire,* The Board of Agriculture, 1802.

Porter, Roy, *The Greatest Benefit to Mankind; a medical history of humanity from antiquity to the present.* London, Fontana Press, 1997.

Raistrick, Arthur, *Dynasty of Ironfounders: the Darbys of Coalbrookdale,* London, Longmans, Green and Co. 1953.

Randall, John., *History of Madeley including Ironbridge, Coalbrookdale and Coalport,* Wrekin Echo Office, Madeley, 1880.

Sandwith, F., *Surgeon Compassionate, the story of Willam Marsden,* Peter Davies, 1960.

Smith, Lance, 'Shropshire in the First Cholera Epidemic', in *Transaction of the Shropshire Archaeological and History Society,* Vol LXXXIV, 2009.

Steggall, John, *A manual for students preparing for examination at Apothecaries Hall or other medical examinations,* London, John Churchill, 1838.

Styrap, Jukes de, *A Code of Medical Ethics,* London, H. K. Lewis, 4th ed., 1895.

Syder, Charles Mingay, *A Series of Questions and Answers for use by gentlemen preparing for their examination at Apothecaries' Hall,* London, Otridge and Rackham, 1823.

Thomas, Emyr, *Coalbrookdale and the Darby Family,* Sessions Book Trust in association with Ironbridge Gorge Museum Trust, York, The Ebor Press, 1999.

Thomas, Emyr, (ed.) *The Private Journal of Adelaide Darby of Coalbrookdale, from 1833 to 1861,* transcribed by Rachel Labouchere, Sessions Book Trust in association with Ironbridge Gorge Museum Trust, York, The Ebor Press, 2004.

Tomkins, Alannah. 'The registers of a provincial man-midwife, Thomas Higgins of Wem 1781-1803', in *Shropshire Historical Documents, a Miscellany,* Shropshire Record Series, Centre for Local History, University of Keele, 2000.

Trinder, Barry, *The Industrial Revolution in Shropshire,* Chichester, Phillimore and Co, 1981.

Trinder, B., in *Shropshire Archaeological Transactions,* Vol lviii, 1965-68, pp 244-258, quoting Hulbert, C. *Hist. Salop, (1837)* ii.

Ward, Conor, *Dr John Langdon Down and Normansfield,* London, Langdon Down Centre Trust, undated.

Watts, S., 'Shifnal Iron Accounts, 1583-90' in *Shropshire Historical Documents, a Miscellany',* Shropshire Record Series, Centre for Local History, University of Keele, 2000, pp12-13.

Archive material

SA, 1987/56/2 to 1987/56/32, Correspondence of the Edwards family of Coalbrookdale, 1814-1838.

SA 1987/64/6, *A Sketch of Coalbrookdale*, manuscript, unsigned and undated.

SA, 2280/6/95, Minutes of Madeley parish council 1780-94.

SA 1987/2/1, Copy Lease, between Rt. Hon. William, Lord Craven, and Benjamin Wright.

SA, 1987/13/3-4, Lease and release — mortgage: Thorpe, Lane, Share and Wright.

Chronology

Benjamin Wright born 26 Mar, at Tattenhall, Cheshire	1745	Stuart uprising in Scotland and England
	1765	James Watt improves steam engines
	1766	Hydrogen discovered by Cavedish
Benjamin Wright marries Fanny Guest	1768	Arkwright's water powered cotton-spinner
		Royal Academy of Arts founded
Mary Wright born (married John Baker)	1770	
Elizabeth Wright born	1771	
Richard Edwards born	1772	Nitrogen discovered by Rutherford
James Wright born, dies young	1774	Oxygen discovered by Priestley
William Edwards born	1775	Watt and Boulton start Soho partnership
Peter Wright born (married Mary Page)	1776	America declares indepence
Benjamin Wright awarded Humane Soc Medal	1777	
	1778	France and Holland allied, Britain declares war
	1779	Spain declares war on Britain
Fanny born	1781	First Iron Bridge opened
	1782	James Watt's double action rotary engine
Rebecca born (married Christopher Bancks)	1784	First purpose built Royal Mail coach runs
	1785	Cartwright invents power loom
	1785	Withering describes medical use of digitalis
	1786	Coal & cotton industries promote economic boom
Anne born (married William Bancks)	1787	Quakers propose abolition of slave trade

	1789	American War of Independence ends
		French revolution begins
Capt Edwards involved in Pandora expedition	1790	
Benjamin Wright leases land for Green Bank	1791	Priestley's house destroyed by rioters
	1792	Coal gas used for lighting
	1792	Corresponding Society founded (electoral reform)
Green Bank occupied	1793	France declares war on Britain
Benjamin dies. Frances to 'hold & occupy' Green Bank	1794	
	1795	Britain declares war on Holland
	1795	Speenhamland wage subsidies
	1795	Severe flood of R Severn
	1795	Poverty and famine in Coalbrookdale
	1795	First iron-framed flax-mill built in Shrewsbury
		Shrewsbury banks fail
William Edwards and **Elizabeth Wright** marry	1796	Poverty persists. Rice distributed
Elizabeth Edwards (Betsey) born	1797	Wordsworth suspected of being a French spy
Edward Edwards born	1798	
	1799	Royal College of Surgeons founded
	1800	Infra-red rays discovered
	1800	Treaty of Amiens between Britain & France
	1803	Dalton proposes atomic theory
Richard Edwards born	1804	Trevethick's first steam train works
	1805	Battle of Trafalgar. Rejoicing in the land
Fanny Edwards born	1807	Gas lighting begins in London

CHRONOLOGY

Anna Maria born	*1809*	George III declared insane
	1811	Luddite movement begins
William Edwards junior born	*1813*	
	1814	First Treaty of Paris, war stops temporarily
Edward's first visit to London	*1814*	Napoleon deposed and exiled to Elba
	1815	Apothecaries Act
Admiral Edwards dies	*1815*	Battle of Waterloo ends European war
Mary Edwards born, dies in infancy	*1815*	Humphry Davy invents Miner's Saftey Lamp
Benjamin Edwards junior born	*1816*	Post-war ecomonic depression
	1819	Peterloo massacre
	1819	Telford builds Menai Straits bridge
Richard Edwards dies aged 20, buried Quaker ground	*1820*	Colliers riot in Coalbrookdale
Anna Maria very ill	*1821*	
Edward Edwards qualifies LSA and MRCS	*1822*	Royal Pavilion Brighton completed (John Nash)
William Edwards junior dies	*1824*	
William Edwards senior dies	*1828*	University and King's Colleges, London, founded
Edward involved in Noden rape case	*1828*	
Anna Maria's sudden return from Cheltenham	*1830*	Cholera epidemic begins
	1830	Ironbridge dispensary opens
	1831	Swing riots affect agriculture
	1831	Charles Darwin sails in HMS Beagle
Rev Richard Edwards dies	*1832*	Cholera epidemic reaches Severn
	1834	Reform Act passed
Anna Maria dies, aged 25	*1834*	Poor Law Amendment Act

189

	1834	First Trades Union formed
	1834	Tolpuddle Martyrs sentenced for joining a trade union
	1835	Charles Babbage designs an early 'computer'
Peter Wright has accident with coach	*1835*	Municipal Corporations Act
Benjamin begins studies in London	*1836*	Chartist movement begins
Edward - Benjamin disagreement	*1836*	Reconstruction work on Rose Hill completed
Benjamin qualifies LSA and MRCS	*1837*	Poor Law Unions in Shropshire defined
	1837	Queen Vicroria succeeds William IV
	1837	Wheatstone and Cooke invent electric telegraph
	1837	Registration of briths, marriages and deaths begins
	1838	Maiden voyage of Brunel's *SS Great Britian*
	1839	Fox Talbot invents photography
	1844	Railway 'mania' 5,000 miles of track completed
	1847	First use of choloroform as anaesthetic
Edward buys Green Bank freehold	*1850*	
	1851	Great Exhibition in London
Fanny dies aged 48	*1855*	
	1858	Medical Act passed: General Medical Council formed
Elizabeth Edwards (mother) dies aged 79	*1858*	Second cholera epidemic
	1859	Darwin publishes *On the Origin of Species*
Benjamin attends Horsehay accident	*1861*	

CHRONOLOGY

Peter Wright dies	*1861*	
	1865	Jospeph Lister introduces antiseptic surgery
	1869	First women's college at Cambridge University
Benjamin moves to Stoney Bank	*1870*	
Edward dies, aged 72	*1871*	New Coalbrookdale church opens
	1871	Trades Unions legalised
	1871	Non-Anglicans admitted to Oxford & Cambridge
	1876	Alexander Graham Bell invents telephone
W H Wright, son of Peter, inherits Green Bank	*1878*	
Betsey dies aged 78	*1878*	
Benjamin dies aged 65	*1881*	First attempt to build Channel Tunnel (fails)

Index

A

Abernethy, John 141
Anatomy 57, 84, 107,
Anglican Church 22, 72
Antimony 16, 20,
Antiseptic 167
Apothecary (ies) 3-7, 14-17, 31-38, 58-62, 77-83, 86- 94, 158-159, 161, 171-173, 180-181
  Act *(1815)* 7, 51, 58, 83, 86, 98, 146, 161-162
  Association 61
  Court of Examiners of the 82, 108, 144
  Hall 108-109, 144, 149
  Society of 51, 59, 61-62, 80-82, 86, 108, 130, 144-145,
  Surgeon 60-62, 80,
Appleby, Susannah 150
Apprenticeship 32-35, 60, 82, 98, 106, 134
Arnott, Dr Neil 159
Association, The British Medical 132
Association, Provincial Medical and Surgical 131, 161-162
Assize (s) 118-121

B

Bailey, George 168-169, 171
Balm of Gilead 17
Bancks,
  Ann 65
  Christopher 187
  William 187
Banks, Dr Thomas 178
Barbados Tar 78
Battle
  of Trafalgar 52, 188
  of Waterloo 76, 189

Bell, Alexander Graham 191
Birkbeck, Dr George 156
Bleeding 94, 152, 167, 181
Bligh, Lieutenant 53
Blistering 16-17
BMA 132, 163-164
Board of Health 122-124
Botany 6, 135, 139
Botfield, William 124
Boulton, Matthew 133
Brande, William 141
Bridgnorth (Shrops) 44
Bristol 131, 158
Britain 2, 9, 13, 15, 21, 53, 69, 85, 87, 99, 122, 127, 131-133, 161, 164, 166, 181
  Railways 51
British Annals of Medicine 86
British Association for the Advancement of Science 130
British Medical Journal, The ix, 162
Brookes, Mr 62, 84, 129
Broseley (Shrops) 2-3, 32, 72, 107, 109, 122, 124, 129, 166
Brougham Henry MP 157

C

Cancer 38, 166, 181
Carpenters Row 42
Certificates 82
Charity Row 42
Chartist (Movement) 86, 103, 127
Chemistry 83-84, 139,
  Pharmaceutical 109
Cholera 122, 124-127, 133, 165
Cinder Hills 101-102
de Cladbrook, Walter 8
Clinical
  Experience 56, 82, 84, 139, 157-158, 160

Studies 160
Coalbrookdale
   Colebrook Dale 10
Coalbrookdale (cont)
   Company 3-5, 42, 44, 46, 50, 71, 73, 103, 116, 164, 176, 180
   Upper Furnace Pool 14, 28-29, 67, 75, 91, 93
   Works 92-93
Coalport 20
Cobbett, William 126, 128
Coke (Coak *sic*) 9, 75, 180
   Production 9, 93
Colebrook Dale *see* Coalbrookdale
Consumption 30, 36, 77, 165-166
Corn Laws 99
Cow Pock 165
Crown and Anchor Tavern 58, 61, 79, 145
Cupping 16-17, 167
Cureton
   Ann 117
   Case 117-118, 133
   Elizabeth 116-121
   Richard 116-117

D

Dance of Death 94
Darby
   Abraham I 29
   Abraham II 29, 44
   Abraham III 18, 20, 22, 24, 29
   Adelaide 152, 173
   Alfred 124
   Deborah 18, 20
   Francis 165
   Maria 152, 166
   Rebecca 29-30, 111
   Richard 152
   Sarah 150
   Road 3, 31
Darwin
   Charles 32, 181

   Robert Dr 24, 32
Davy, Sir Humphry 6-7, 73, 133
Dawley
   Board 124
   Parish 124, 129, 176
   Parish Council 124
Diseases
   Erysipelas 37, 42
   Heart 87, 166
   Paget's 35
   Respiratory 36, 87
   Skin 38
   Smallpox 39
   Venereal 37, 120
Dispensary 56, 107, 139, 148, 157
Dissection 34, 56, 136, 139
Down, John Langdon Dr 35

E

Edinburgh 35, 114
Education, Medical 6, 34, 51-53, 88, 118, 135, 143, 146-147, 149, 154, 158, 161,
Edwards
   Anna Maria 48-49, 70, 99, 110-111, 133, 134
   Benjamin 1, 5 *et al*
   Captain Edward (RN) 34, 53,
   Edward 1, 6-7 *et al*
   Elizabeth (neé Wright) 5, 27, 30, 31-33, 40-41, 47-48 63-64, 70, 103-106, 110, 113, 134, 152, 172-174
   Fanny 99, 109-113, 133, 134, 152, 172-174, 179
   Mary 5, 27, 48, 70, 114
   Richard 31, 55, 134
   William 1, 5 *et al*
Elixir Paregoric 20
Epsom Salts 167
Erysipelas *see* Disease
Extracts of Colchicine 137
Ex Hyosc 137

INDEX

F
Faraday, Michael 6, 133, 180
Farr, William 86
Fletcher, Rev John 52, 72, 74
Flood 40, 44-45, 75
France 2, 4-5, 85-87
Frost Fairs 45, 63-64

G
General Medical Council 132, 163
General Pharmaceutical Association 59
General Practitioner 62, 81-83, 98, 148, 153, 163, 165-166
Gower Street 157
Great
    Meeting 79, 145-146
    Reform Act 127, 143
Green Bank Farm 29
Greenbank (House) 5, 175, 177
Guest
    Charles 32
    Frances, 5, 27, 31, 33, 65, 70
    John 3, 32

H
Halford, Sir Henry 158
Harrison, Dr Edward 60
Hastings, Charles 130
Hewison Ann (of Godmanchester) 34
Higgins, Thomas 18, 21
HMS Bounty 53
HMS Pandora 53
Holy Trinity Church (Coalbrookdale) 173, 177
Humane Society 21-22
Hunterian Oration 148

I
Iron Bridge 4, 44, 46, 68 72, 92, 129, 149 164, 180

Gorge Museum 92-93, 96, 180
Ironmasters 3, 14, 48, 93, 101, 124

J
Jenner, Edward 39

L
Labouchere, Lady Rachel xi
Laennec, Richard 87-88, 96
Lancet, The 35, 131, 136, 144-146, 149, 152, 162
Langdon Down, Dr John 35, 66
Lawley Bank 19, 101
Lawrence, William 141
Lightmoor 41, 47, 176
Lister, Joseph 167
Little Dawley 27, 43
Little Wenlock 39, 43, 52, 109, 178
Loamhole Brook 29
London
    Board of Health 122-123
    Society of Apothecaries 51, 61, 81
    University 135, 147, 154, 156-157, 160
Loxham, Dr 37-38

M
Madeley 9, 14, 72, 74
    Parish Council 22
    Union of Parishes 128-129
Madeley (cont)
    Wood 11, 19, 46
Malinslee 72, 112, 173
Man-midwife 95, 105, 107
Manchester 158, 164
    Patriotic Union 100
Marsden, William 35, 66
Medical
    Act 8, 132, 146, 156, 162-163, 171, 172
    Education *see* Education

Ethics 121, 133, 170
Register 8, 132, 163, 171
Students 7, 34, 51, 143-146, 157, 160, 163
Medicines Act 59
Medical Times and Gazette, The 116, 176, 178
Medico-Ethical Associations 171
Much Wenlock 8, 118
Municipal
    Boroughs Act 127
    Corporations Acts 86, 143, 161

N

Nailers Row 42
Napoleon 40, 76, 137
National Health Service 45, 76, 128, 181
National Insurance 181
Noden, John 117-122
Norfolk 112, 174-175

O

Origin of Species 181

P

Paget, Sir James MD 35
Palin, Thomas 102
Parish of Madeley *see* Madeley
Peel, Robert 120-121
Penny Post 12, 79, 131
Percival, Thomas 36, 170
Peterloo Massacre 85, 100-101, 143
Pharmacopoeia Londonensis 109
Poor
    House 23, 30
    Law 123, 128-129
    Amendment Act 128
    Commission 128-129
Priestley, Joseph 102, 133
Privy Council 122-123
Provincial Medical Practitioners of England 131
Pulsford 36-38

Q

Quaker 3, 5, 22, 29, 44, 71-73, 76, 98, 112
Friends 72
Meeting House 71

R

Radcliffe, Dr 17
Rheumatic 77, 151
Rhubarb Hall 145
Riot Act 101
River Severn 3-4, 8, 11, 43-44, 122
River Thames 45, 63-64, 70, 105, 138
Rose Hill 5, 31, 33, 42, 48, 70-71, 91, 93, 97, 110, 117, 134, 150, 172, 174-176
Rosehill 3, 5, 28-29

Royal
    College of Physicians 35, 59-60, 78, 80, 130, 158
    Surgeons 35, 80, 130, 139, 148, 156, 159, 162
    Free Hospital 35
    Humane Society 21-22
    Institution 7
    Marsden Hospital 35

S

Salop Infirmary 37, 42, 178
Salopian Journal 127, 162
School House Row 42
Severn Gorge 8, 180
Seward, Anna 10, 93, 180
Shifnal 14, 68, 70

Shrewsbury 71, 102, 104, 107, 118-119, 122-123, 126, 131-132, 162
   Assize 118
   Bank 46
   Borough Corporation 123
   Chronicle 126
Sick Club 47
Small Pox 165
Smith, Thomas 143-146, 154
Smokey Row 42
Snow, Dr John 127
Sorton, Ann 152
Stamp Duty 59
Steggal (*Manual for Students*) 154-155
Stoney Hill 176, 178-179
Styrap 170
Surgeon Apothecary see Apothecary
Sydenham, Dr Thomas, Dr 54

T

Tea Kettle Row 91, 116-117
Telford 9, 14, 176
Telford, Thomas 44
Thakrah, William 36
The Chestnuts 150
The Old Incline 176
Tooth Instruments 65
Trevithick, Richard 50, 96, 133, 180
Turner, Thomas 21
Typhus 30, 37, 111-112, 134, 151-153, 165-166, 174

U

Union Medical Officers 129, 131, 162
University
   College Hospital 157
   of London 135, 147, 157, 160
Upper Furnace Pool 14, 28-29, 67, 75, 91, 93
Upper Works 93

V

Vaughan, Sir John 118, 121
Voluntary Subscription Hospitals 57

W

Wakley, Thomas 35, 146
Walters, Constable 118
Warburton, Henry 146
Watt, James 7
Wellington 15, 71, 152,
   Journal 169
Western General Dispensary 107
Wilkinson, John 4, 46
Withering, William 15
Wolverhampton 10, 164
Worcester 68, 130-131
Worcester (cont)
   Infirmary 131
Wright,
   Ann 31
   Benjamin 1, 5 *et al*
   Elizabeth 5, 27, 30, 31-33, 40-41, 47-49, 63-64, 70, 103-106, 110, 113, 134, 152, 172-174
   Peter 5, 31-32, 65, 103, 117, 119-121, 125, 173, 175, 177
   Sarah 107
   William Henry 177

Y

Yate 41, 65, 104
   Joseph 178-179
Yorkshire Philosophical Society 130
Young, Arthur 10